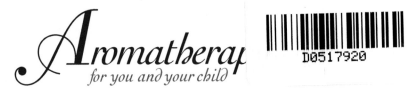

Aromatherap

for you and your child

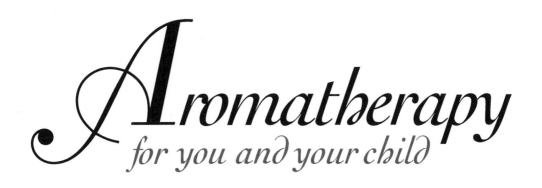

Aromatherapy
for you and your child

By **Tara Fellner**

Illustrations by **Betsy James**

CHARLES E. TUTTLE COMPANY, INC.
Boston • Rutland, Vermont • Tokyo

This book is dedicated to Kristine Weaver Dunn, my aromatic partner and friend, whose patience, good nature, and tireless devotion to our mutual cause makes anything possible.

First published in 1995 by Charles E. Tuttle Co., Inc.
of Rutland, Vermont and Tokyo, Japan, with editorial offices
at 153 Milk Street, Boston, Massachusetts 02109

ISBN 0-8048-3043-6

Design by Learning Arts Publications

Illustrations by Betsy James

3 5 7 9 10 8 6 4 2   02 01 00 99 98 97 96 95

Printed in the United States

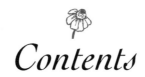

Contents

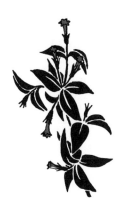

Preface and Acknowledgments

May you live in interesting times.
CHINESE CURSE

I don't know about you, but when I look at the era in which I am raising my children, a bit of Dickens from my junior high school literature class comes to mind: "It was the best of times, it was the worst of times." Women have made impressive strides in the areas of basic civil liberties and professional and economic opportunity in the last hundred years. We are free to vote, to own property, to be educated, to rise to the highest levels of any profession we choose. Where the glass ceiling still exists, there are so many women pounding on it from beneath that we feel confident it will eventually shatter, if not for us, then surely for our daughters who come after us.

Our gains, however, have not come unaccompanied by losses. For many of us, economic and professional freedom means working full- or part-time in addition to maintaining the responsibilities of a home and family. The frenetic pace of modern motherhood subjects women to higher levels of stress, which leave us vulnerable to an ever-increasing host of stress-related disorders. Our children are suffering too. Yet, as is often the case, what produces the cause also produces the cure. The same technological approach that has created environmental imbalances on a global scale has also globally linked us all. We now have at our fingertips precious essences from all over the world, once solely within reach of rulers and the very rich.

Like fragrant breaths of Paradise, essential oils help reconnect us to the natural world that is our true home. While they can, as you will discover, be used to treat the symptoms of illness, the essences are most often used holistically by aromatherapists, with a focus on healing the whole person rather than treating a particular disease. As breakthroughs in medical research make us more aware of how the body operates, we begin to get a sense of the intricate connections that link thought, emotion, stress levels, and immune function. Used knowledgeably and responsibly, essential oils help to calm the mind, balance the emotions, heal the body, and uplift the spirit. All these things are necessary for us to experience a vibrant level of health.

Motherhood is a sacred privilege and each child born is a treasure to be opened with love—protected, respected, and admired. This is my belief. Through the practice of aromatherapy we can use essential oils as keys to a richer, healthier, and more pleasurable experience of life. It is in this spirit that I offer this introductory guide to their use, with the profound wish that you and your children will discover the magic of aromatherapy and benefit by it as my children and I have.

Included with this kit are several preblended bath and massage products that are produced by wives tales, a company I cofounded. The formulas for these products were developed through aromatherapy experiences with my own children, Nick and Margaret, now eight and four years of age, respectively. I hope that you and your children will enjoy using them!

I give heartfelt thanks to Michael Kerber of Charles E. Tuttle Co., Inc., and Ron Schultz, Terry Duffy, and "the gang" at Learning Arts for this opportunity to share with other families what I've learned. I deeply appreciate Eugenia Melissaratos for sharing her love and knowledge of essential oils and Tara Kamath for contributing the benefits of her extensive experience with essential oils and massage. Teresa Ramsey provided valuable insight on the art of baby massage. For computer assistance I am indebted to John Scandurra. Jane Kennedy and the "Palmetto girls" are a continuous source of inspiration and support. Debra Kay and Greg Evans, Carol Corio, Ellie Garber, Pam Gillis, Alison McDaniel, Amy Weber, and Edna Lucia Lopez, none of it would happen without you! To my mother, Marlene Fellner, my bonus set of parents, John and Lois Haugner, and world-class sweetie Paul Shabazian, thanks for your love and emotional support. I am truly blessed to know you all.

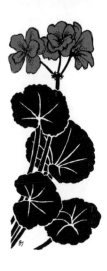

Chapter One

AROMATHERAPY: WHAT IT IS AND HOW IT WORKS

Come forth into the Light of Things,
Let Nature be your teacher.

WILLIAM WORDSWORTH

For tens of thousands of years, aromatic plants have been in common use for a multitude of purposes. They have been used to preserve meat and embalm human flesh, to prevent and cure diseases, to influence mood, and to seduce. Incenses and perfumes carried the prayers of our ancestors to their gods, and almost all primitive peoples share the common beliefs that good smells attract good spirits and a beautiful fragrance is a breath of the Divine.

We women carry deep associations with the world of plants. After all, we invented agriculture, and we may have invented the distillation process that was crucial to the development of aromatherapy as well. While the credit for inventing distillation has long been given to Avicenna, a tenth-century Arab physician, there exists a drawing of a still invented by Maria Prophetissima, an alchemist from Alexandria, that predates Avicenna's by centuries.

During the Early Paleolithic period, when the first human beings (*Homo habilis*) appeared, an almost instantaneous division of labor took place that would subsequently influence the social and cultural development of the species. Men became hunters, and women turned to botany, adding variety to the dinner table and staying close enough to home to raise their slow-growing offspring. This arrangement allowed for the evolution of more powerful, postnatally developed brains and the eventual proliferation of our species all over the planet. And still, countless centuries later, when, gardening, I put my hands into the earth, I experience a deep calm. Of course! It's only natural. I am repeating a gesture women have been making for two and a half million years.

But lest we get too great a sense of our own importance in the planetary scheme of things, it's humbling to remember that the age of the Earth is estimated at some 4,500 million years. We are relative newcomers here. Aromatic plants have been with the planet much longer than we have. Terpenes, the first aromatic molecules, appeared with the conifers about three hundred million years ago, with flowers following a hundred million years later, at roughly the same time that dinosaurs came to dominate the still-shifting continents. It would be another hundred million years before our mammal foremothers even developed the placenta.

And so, when you open and sniff a vial of pine essential oil, you invite into your body molecules that have existed more than 297 million years longer than your oldest ancestor. With a drop of rose, hundred-million-year-old molecules enter your bloodstream and course through your veins. Quite apart from the more obvious benefits to health and well-being, aromatherapeutic use of essential oils allows you to connect with the earth at a molecular level, in a deep and primordial way.

Most of the process that establishes our olfactory circuits takes place during early childhood. There is evidence that the human fetus may begin using the sense of smell while still in the womb. Infants have been shown to recognize the smell of their mothers within ten minutes following birth. The emotional connections that anchor our smell memories during these formative phases of development will be deeply ingrained in our nervous systems, with tremendous power to influence us throughout life. To one writer, the smell of tobacco that lingered on his father's fingers was the smell of love, and Charles Dickens was plunged into the depths of despair by the odor of glue, which brought with it all the anguish and feelings of abandonment he experienced as a young boy when his destitute father deserted him in a bottle factory.

What were the smells of your childhood? What will your children remember? Conscious and aware use of essential oils for purposes of aromatherapy can create wonderful "smell memories" for you and your child. Think about the fragrances you'd like your child to associate with your love and attention, at bathtime, at bedtime, during quiet times you share together. These early associations will be with both of you for life, as you deepen the healing partnership that has existed between human beings and the plant world since the dawn of human history.

Modern Aromatherapy

Modern aromatherapy is generally recognized as originating with the man who coined the term back in the 1900s and published several books on the subject, a French cosmetic chemist by the name of René Maurice Gattefosse. Born in the province of Lyons in 1881, Gattefosse was the son of a perfumer and became fascinated with the use of essential oils as popular medicines among the peasants who worked the lavender fields. Following an explosion in his laboratory in 1910, he successfully used the healing and cell-regenerating properties of lavender essential oil on his own severely burned hands and scalp. Impressed by the results, he embarked on a series of investigations into essential oils and their medicinal properties, publishing his findings in several books. He also created products based on his research, such as an essential oil-based antiseptic soap he formulated to help halt the progress of the deadly Spanish flu epidemic of 1918. Working in association with army doctors, veterinarians, and hospitals, Gattefosse continued to test applications for his essential oil formulas until his death in Casablanca in 1950. His investigations helped form much of the basis of modern aromatherapy, especially as currently practiced medically in Europe.

During World War II, army surgeon Dr. Jean Valnet, who was influenced by Gattefosse, confirmed the healing properties of many essential oils that he used under the extreme conditions of wartime surgery when supplies of penicillin ran short. Valnet continued his research into both medical and psychiatric uses for the essences after the war and in 1964 published his book *Aromatherapy*, a fascinating and informative text on

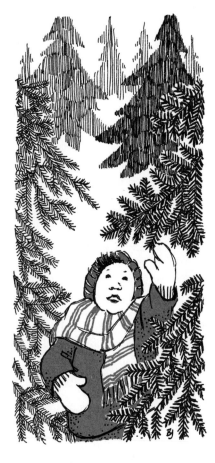

medical applications of essential oils. He began to teach aromatherapy to medical doctors in his native France, and there are now several thousand medical practitioners who prescribe essential oils in Europe. Prominent among them is the notable French physician Daniel Penoel, whose clinical work with essential oils puts him at the forefront of modern medical aromatherapy.

Marguerite Maury, a French biochemist and contemporary of Dr. Valnet, researched the effects of essential oils used in conjunction with massage and was awarded the Prix International for her discoveries. Other women responsible for groundbreaking work in the aromatherapy field include Micheline Arcier, Daniele Ryman, Patricia Davis, Valerie Worwood, and Shirley Price.

Robert Tisserand is generally recognized as being almost single-handedly responsible for the surge of popular interest in aromatherapy as a result of his several excellent books on the subject. Interesting research is currently being conducted by Dr. Daniel Lapraz, Pierre Franchomme, and American archaeologist John Steele.

To understand essential oils and their benefits more fully, let's begin by defining what, for purposes of aromatherapy, essential oils are and how they are used.

Essential Oils

Essential "oils" are not really oils at all but fragrant, highly concentrated, chemically complex essences extracted from aromatic plant material such as flowers, stems, leaves, roots, barks, fruits, seeds, and resins. On average, an essential oil is 70 to 100 times more concentrated than fresh or dried plant material alone. When used for purposes of aromatherapy, the essences are inhaled with the breath or applied to the skin. Because the molecules are so small and are by nature lipophilic, or attracted to the fats in the outer layers of the skin, essential oils are easily absorbed into the body, thereby entering the bloodstream and circulating for several hours before being excreted with sweat, urine, or breath. By contrast, the larger molecules of herbs and tinctures are up to 100 times slower to penetrate.

In Europe, where aromatherapy is practiced by many doctors and nurses, and where essential oils are available in pharmacies, the essences may be prescribed for internal use. This practice is **not advised** without the guidance of a qualified medical practitioner, as some essential oils can cause liver damage when used over extended periods. In the United States, the essences are most often used through external applications such as massage, baths, or skin care, which will be described in more detail in the following chapters.

All essential oils are antiseptic and antibacterial to a degree, depending on their dominant chemical constituents. Their healing properties are determined in part by their botanical family. For instance, the Labiatae, which includes lavender, thyme, rosemary, and sage, tend to be strong antiseptics with cicatrizing properties, which makes them excellent choices for the cleansing and healing of wounds. (For a full recounting of essential oils by botanical family, see Marcel Lavabre's *Aromatherapy Workbook*.)

Essences are chemically characterized by the presence of carbon-based terpenoid compounds such as terpene alcohols, aldehydes, ketones, esters, and ethers. The terpenoid compounds affect the basic metabolism of the bacteria. To live, a cell must breathe. All its life energy is generated by respiration, during which it produces a metabolic chemical known as ATP. When an essential oil gets into a bacteria's cell membrane, it inhibits production of ATP and may also literally smother the bacteria by cutting off its respiration. This explains why bacteria don't become resistant to treatment with essential oils over time, as is common with the use of pharmaceutical drugs such as antibiotics. Any living thing that depends on breathing for its life force will have a tough time developing resistance to being smothered!

Dominant chemical constituents will also affect the way in which an essential oil is used therapeutically. Lavender, dominated by soothing, balancing esters, promotes relaxation and eases stress. Ketones are mucolytic: they slow down the production of mucous, and their strong presence in eucalyptus essential oil explains why it has been used the world over to relieve respiratory congestion. High aldehyde content tends to make an oil that is calming and anti-inflammatory as well as antiseptic, such as lemongrass and the nearly impossible to obtain true melissa. (For a detailed explanation of the chemistry of essential oils, see Dr. Kurt Schnaubelt's Aromatherapy course listed in the Resource Guide.)

Properly chosen and applied, essential oils are very safe to use and cause virtually no side effects. As aggressive as the essences are toward pathogenic organisms, they remain harmless to the tissue that harbors the invaders. Many essential oils are used in skin care to promote new cell growth and retard the aging process. In addition, aromatics produce noticeable effects on mood and emotion, which can in turn influence bodily functions.

The study of the effects of fragrance on mood and emotion is called "aromachology," a term coined by Annette Green of the Fragrance Foundation. Aromachology, while related to aromatherapy, differs in that the fragrances employed can be of synthetic or natural origin. In aromatherapy, only pure, whole essential oils are used.

The use of pure, distilled aromatic essences is also what differentiates aromatherapy from herbalism and other plant-based healing modalities. Essential oils are extracted from aromatic plants by one of the following methods.

WATER OR STEAM DISTILLATION

This is the method by which many of the most commonly used essential oils, such as lavender, rosemary, eucalyptus, and peppermint, are obtained. Steam is infused through plant material, rupturing tiny sacs between plant cells that hold the aromatic essence. The steam carries the essence away and is cooled and condensed in a separate chamber. The essential oil is then skimmed off the surface of the water. This results in a very pure essence considered safe for use on the human body (depending, of course, on the oil chosen and how it is applied). Inorganic compounds that would be

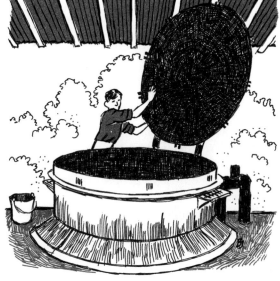

incompatible with human biochemistry, such as pesticides and contaminants, tend to be left behind in the plant matter.

The aromatic water that is a by-product of the distillation process may contain beneficial elements from the plant material as well and is often used in skin care as a toner or facial spray or as an ingredient in soaps or lotions. Popular floral waters include rose, neroli (also known as orange blossom), lavender, and chamomile.

COLD PRESSING

Also known as "expression," this method utilizes pressure to extract the volatile oils from the peelings of citrus fruits. Orange, tangerine, lemon, lime, bergamot, and mandarin are examples of essential oils obtained by cold pressing.

CO₂ DISTILLATION

CO_2 distillation methods have been used since the late 1800s to refine and extract a variety of substances, from fractionating crude oil to extracting the lanolin from wool fat and decaffeinating coffee.

For production of essential oils, pressurized carbon dioxide replaces steam as the catalyst for breaking down plant matter in the distillation process. This method is used for spice oils, such as black pepper, ginger, and nutmeg, and is extremely useful for distilling delicate aromatics that tend to break down or change in character when heat is applied. CO_2 is a cleaner alternative to solvent methods, which tend to leave a residue of petrochemicals in the finished product.

This method produces a very "true" smelling essence, that is, the essential oil smells almost identical to the aromatic plant from which it comes. CO_2 can also be used to create "whole plant" extracts that contain more elements of the plant material than just the essential oil. For example, the healing properties of calendula flowers, which do not produce an essential oil per se, can be extracted this way. Carbon dioxide distillation has also been used to produce a total extraction of marjoram that contains more of the healing benefits of the whole herb but in highly concentrated form.

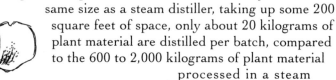

CO_2 distillations may be a little pricier as essential oils go, since less essence is produced per batch. While the machinery is about the same size as a steam distiller, taking up some 200 square feet of space, only about 20 kilograms of plant material are distilled per batch, compared to the 600 to 2,000 kilograms of plant material processed in a steam

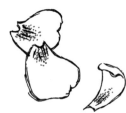

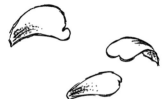

distillation. Essential oil yield from the plant material distilled is about 3 percent or less by weight. For rare and precious oils such as helichrysm, the yield can be as little as $^2/_{10}$ of a percent.

SOLVENT EXTRACTION

Certain flowers, such as jasmine, produce minute amounts of exquisite essences too fragile to press or distill yet too beautiful to be allowed to disappear completely with the last breath of spring. These delicate scents may be preserved for continued enjoyment by extraction through fatty or chemical solvents. The essence is then separated from the solvent, leaving a waxy substance known as a concrete. Further purification of the concrete using alcohol and carefully monitored heat will yield an absolute. Essences obtained by solvent extraction tend to be used more for their fragrance and perfume applications, since solvent residue may render them inappropriate for aromatherapeutic purposes.

Enfleurage, an ancient method that involves placing layers of fragrant petals on panels smeared with fat, is still used in the production of tuberose absolute. When their aroma has migrated into the fat, the spent petals are removed and replaced with fresh blossoms. When the desired concentration has been achieved, the essence is then separated from the fat.

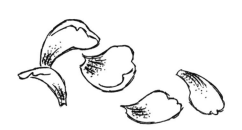

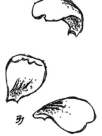

This is a method used to remove any traces of solvent residue from delicate essences, such as rose, that have been solvent-extracted. High vacuum distillation creates an extremely pure essential oil with a fragrance that is very true to the flower.

More About Essential Oils

Essential oils for individual use are sold in small, dark glass bottles that range in size from a few milliliters for precious oils to the more common one-third- or one-half-ounce sizes (about 10 and 15 ml respectively). Prices vary widely and fluctuate according to variables such as rarity of the oil, size of that year's harvest, and the therapeutic potency of the essence, which will be determined by its chemical composition, which is in turn determined by factors such as soil composition, where it was grown, what the weather was like during the growing season, and how and when the plant material was harvested.

Bottles of essential oil should be kept tightly capped when not in use, since many of the oils are highly volatile and will evaporate when exposed to air. Many essential oils can retain their aromas and healing properties for years if properly stored away from heat and sunlight. A reputable supplier will include on the bottle's label the botanical name of the plant from which the essence was distilled and possibly the country of origin as well.

Knowing the exact botanical name of an essential oil is important when choosing an oil such as eucalyptus, of which some three hundred botanical varieties exist, at least ten of which are available as essential oils, each with its own particular application in aromatherapy. *Eucalyptus globulus* is a "standard"-smelling eucalyptus commonly used for respiratory conditions, while *E. citriodora* has an intense lemony smell and is generally used for other purposes, such as repelling insects.

Aromatherapists tend to think of the oils as living essences, describing them as the "soul" or "life force" of a plant. An essential oil may also be thought of as integral to a plant's "immune system" since more volatile oil tends to be produced by a plant in response to stress from a harsh environment. Some of the most important oil-producing plants grow best under stressful conditions—hot sun, poor soil, little water. Certain plants can be very finicky about where and how they will grow and may produce a superior grade of oil only at a particular altitude or in one very specific part of the world.

Each essence possesses a distinctive aroma, which a sensitive nose can be trained to recognize. But even the most discerning nose can't always tell the difference between an authentic oil and one that has been altered. For purposes of aromatherapy, the intact essential oil, just as it was distilled from the plant, is preferred. In such an oil, the full array of chemical components is believed to work in synergy in a way that has a greater life force and healing potential than an oil that has been tampered with or altered in some way.

An intact essential oil contains trace amounts of mysterious substances, some of which may occur nowhere else in nature and many of which haven't even been named yet. Essential oil of mandarin contains up to 95 percent limonene, an antiviral component, yet many of its healing properties are due to the remaining 5 percent, which contains more than seventy-four identified minor and trace components. A natural rose essence is extremely complex chemically and contains as many as two thousand constituent parts, each of which is necessary to create the fullness of one of Nature's finest aromas and to pack the broad spectrum of healing applications into every drop. Aromatherapists believe that a whole, naturally occurring essential oil has superior potency due to trace constituents that provide a balance to the more obviously active constituents, perhaps lessening irritation or other side effects that would occur if individual components were used in isolation.

Holistic Aromatherapy

The preference for intact essential oils is an extension of the basic concept of "holism" that is central to the practice of true aromatherapy. The holistic approach requires that the whole person must be considered as the context within which a specific symptom occurs.

It's not enough merely to eliminate a symptom if the cause has not been addressed. In holistic thinking, the symptom is viewed as a kind of distress signal, a physical flare of sorts, sent up by the body to get the attention of the mind. "Dis-ease" then becomes more than just a momentary breakdown in the body/machine—it's an attempt made by the body to communicate with the self regarding some kind of imbalance. The suppression of a symptom, if deeper healing has not taken place, will generally result in the appearance of another symptom as the body continues to send up flares. We tend to describe certain recurrent patterns of symptoms as "flare-ups."

The word holism is also related to the concept of "holiness," as it recognizes that the essence of life from which true health derives is, by nature, sacred. We are all sacred beings. Life, in its truest and deepest sense, is a celebration of holiness.

This is a fundamentally different concept from conventional Western medicine, which tends to view medical treatment in more mechanical, even adversarial terms: "attacking" a symptom, "conquering" a disease, "fighting" germs, "battling" epidemics. The underlying idea of holism is that if the system is functioning harmoniously, all its parts will naturally work at optimal capacity. A balanced, healthy system is by nature resistant to disease.

Abundant research published over the past few decades affirms the body/mind connection and its effect on health and well-being. Prayer has been shown to speed the healing process, and what we eat influences not only our physical makeup but our mental clarity, emotions, and mood. Lifestyle and community ties have an impact on the incidence of heart disease. How, and how often, we are touched as children will determine important aspects of our biochemistry, which in turn will influence how we think, what we feel, and how we behave. Changes in any area of our lives, or lifestyles, can have a major impact on our health as a whole.

Essential oils are perfectly suited to the holistic approach because they work simultaneously on many levels to balance and heal. Along with the sense of pleasure stirred by their aromas in the "pleasure center" of the brain and their antiviral, antibacterial, antifungal, and antiseptic properties, certain essential oils can alter the pH level of the blood and change its electrical conductivity within minutes of having been absorbed into the body. On other levels, studies indicate that certain fragrances can influence mood and behavior quite dramatically, for example, causing shoppers to spend more and gamblers to tuck more quarters into slot machines. Aromatherapy is in active use in Japan to improve worker productivity and reduce stress. Specially designed climate control systems there diffuse essences through the air-conditioning ducts of office buildings and factories. Hospitals and hotels in the United States are experimenting with environmental fragrancing for both aesthetic and healthful purposes.

Once you've acquired a basic working knowledge of essential oils and their traditional applications as outlined in the following chapters, don't be afraid to experiment and to use your intuition! Often your body will know what's right for it. Given a variety of choices, choose an oil that smells good and intuitively feels right to you. Recent studies indicate that smell preferences exist for a reason: the aroma you prefer is the one you need.

It takes time and effort to develop a sense of inner knowing regarding our own health and that of our children. If you or your child is seriously ill, by all means seek treatment from a qualified medical practitioner. But don't be afraid to try using aromatherapy on its own or in conjunction with other therapies. Try starting small, using essential oils for everyday problems, to ease a runny nose, take the itch out of a mosquito bite, or promote relaxation at bedtime. Notice and keep a record of which oils work best for you and your family, which conditions respond to them. If the oil you've chosen doesn't seem to be working, try another with similar therapeutic effects, or try decreasing the dosage (odd as it sounds, this works!).

Train your nose with the best oils you can find. Quality essential oils are cheaper in the long run, as a few drops of a high-grade essence can outperform whole bottles of inferior oils. Organic essential oils or essences obtained through responsible wild-crafting are the best, not only because of the lack of pesticide residue but also because the plants that produce them tend to be healthier and stronger and their cultivation has less negative impact on the Earth.

The better you know your oils and the more experience you have using them, the more confident you'll become. Careful and persistent observation can yield volumes of useful information and often makes it possible to nip an imbalance in the bud, rather than waiting for it to turn into a major health problem.

Please remember that aromatherapy, like any treatment, will not be effective 100 percent of the time against any and all complaints. The great challenge and joy of life is that every day is different, every person is unique, and no two situations are ever quite the same. When it comes to maintaining health and well-being, aromatherapy is one tool in a very large toolbox. A hammer is not better than a screwdriver, and while it can be used for a variety of purposes, it can't be used for everything. Likewise, there are instances in which other therapies might be more appropriate. In an emergency situation such as a car accident, a bottle of lavender may be useful to help the victim calm down a bit, but it won't stitch up a gash. (Although you'd certainly want to use it to speed healing and to rebalance after getting the bill from that emergency room visit!) Aromatherapy does not eliminate the need for Western medicine or the family doctor. But I have found that the use of essential oils has definitely cut down on the number of our office visits and lessened the intensity and severity of illnesses when we experience them.

If you follow the guidelines for selection and dosage, it's hard to make a serious mistake. The oils described in this book, and those used in the formulations for the products that accompany it, have been preselected for their safety and effectiveness with women and children.

So go ahead. Experiment! Enjoy! Nature's fragrant healing gems await your discovery.

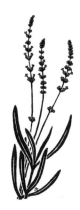

Chapter Two

LAVENDER:
THE STORY OF AN
ESSENTIAL OIL

Lavender is a member of the botanical family Labiatae, which produces many other wonderful aromatic plants whose essences are used in aromatherapy, such as rosemary and clary sage. Like many other healing herbs, lavender was first selected and gathered as a medicinal untold centuries ago from amid the wild, primeval profusion of plant life that once carpeted Europe. Lavender is native to the Mediterranean and grows wild in southern France, Spain, Italy, Corsica, and Sicily. The plant prefers dry, stony land with plenty of sun and will not thrive in low, moist places or tolerate cold winters. Pilgrim John Josselyn discovered this for himself when he tried to duplicate his English garden in the New World, finally concluding, that "Lavender is not for the climate."

Lavender is by far the most often used aromatherapy essential oil, because of the universal appeal of its fragrance and the broad spectrum of its healing applications. Gattefosse originally became interested in the healing properties of essential oils through the use and study of lavender, as did countless other aromatherapy devotees, from Dr. Valnet to Pierre Franchomme to your humble author. I can't begin to count how many little bottles of lavender I have given as gifts or pressed upon dubious friends and family members, only to have them tell me afterward in amazement, "It really works!" Mosquito bites, fevers, pimples, stress, sunburn, insomnia—these are only a few of the conditions that can be eased through the application of lavender essential oil. In fact, it's difficult to think of any condition that can't be helped, if not

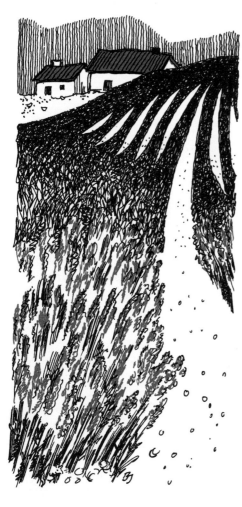

healed, by use of this amazing essence, singly or in combination with other essential oils.

The south of France has been famous for its lavender for centuries and is generally recognized for producing the best lavender essence in the world. French lavender is a perennial plant that blooms with majestic stalks of fragrant purple blossoms each summer for six or seven years, the best yields being produced in the third and fourth years. Recently, lavender growers have been alarmed to find that some of their plants are spent after as little as two years. They link the shortened life span to overall genetic weakening of the plant strain and depletion of the soil caused by the use of pesticides. The good news is that this sobering discovery is leading some growers to return to more natural methods of cultivation. The bad news is that the already small supply of authentic lavender essence may get even smaller, especially with increasing demand worldwide.

More than six hundred years ago, in 1371, wild lavender was first cultivated in the Bourgogne area of France. To this day that once-wild variety is designated as the "true" lavender, known by its botanical name *Lavandula vera* or *L. officinalis*, the "official" lavender of France. Some fifteen subspecies are used in the production of essential oils, from *Lavandula officinalis fragrans*, the wild lavender that grows in very dry limestone soil at an elevation of 2,200 to 5,500 feet, to *L. o. delphinensis*, which will grow in cooler soils at lower elevations. *L. spica*, or spike lavender, has a natural camphor content that makes it particularly useful for respiratory ailments and friction rubs for muscle aches and pains.

Lavandins, such as *Lavandula hybrida abrialis*, *L. h. grosso*, *L. h. Reydovan*, and *L. h. super* are actually hybrids between true lavender and spike lavender, possessing certain properties of both. Lavandins can be useful for situations in which some of the healing properties of lavender are desired without the calming or sleep-inducing qualities. The variety of available lavenders and hybrids again points up the importance of knowing the botanical name and origin of an essential oil, as each subspecies will differ slightly in aroma and therapeutic application.

The Latin name *Lavandula* is derived from the word *lavare*, meaning "to wash," attesting to the fact that long before it was cultivated, distilled, or even named, lavender was in common use for cleansing purposes. The Romans used lavender to perfume their baths, and it is mentioned by the ancient Roman naturalist Pliny and the Greek physician Galen as a tonic and stimulant. The "spikenard" mentioned in the Bible is believed actually to have been lavender, the biblical name having been taken from Nardus, a town in Syria, and "spike," descriptive of the blooming flowers. In Tuscany, lavender protects children from the evil eye, while Kabyle women of North Africa use it to protect themselves from maltreatment by their husbands.

Of the many varieties of lavender available, the official French *Lavandula officinalis* or *L. vera* plant grown in Provence produces the most prized essential oil. Perfumers treasure it for its fine fragrance, aromatherapists for its chemical complexity and superior therapeutic qualities. But only so much of it can be grown in a season. Lavender growers, like most growers of essential oil crops, tend to be hardworking people, often with families, who live simply and frugally, close to the land. A typical small producer of lavender in the south of France might have some twenty hectares (the equivalent of about forty acres), not necessarily adjacent to each other, on which lavender is either growing wild or being cultivated. Most likely the producer's holdings will not be devoted entirely to *L. vera*. As many as five different varieties of lavender are likely to be growing there, which may include the hybridized lavandins and the strain known as English lavender, or maillot.

The annual yield for *L. vera* is comparatively small—about ten kilograms of distilled essential oil produced per acre of lavender plants grown. The yield for the hybrid lavandins can be considerably greater—as high as forty kilograms per acre. Often a small producer's entire crop yield is purchased in advance by large essential oil brokerage houses. Consequently, it's no surprise that somewhere along the line the essential oils produced by the more prolific lavandins and hybrids are likely to be mixed with *L. vera* to stretch the yield. Some sources estimate that up to 98 percent of commercially available essential oils have been adulterated to a greater or lesser degree.

Once the purple blossoms have begun to open, wild lavender is harvested from the mountainside by hand. Cultivated crops are generally cut with the assistance of tractors. The fragrant stalks are then bunched and stacked, ready for distillation. Most likely the producer will not own a distillation unit but will lease time to distill with several other producers of lavender or a similar crop, such as clary sage. A distillation vat may hold thousands of kilograms of plant material and is heated up from below by igniting dried, exhausted plant material, from which the essential oils have already been removed in previous distillations. Distillation time for a full vat of lavender is less than an hour.

Essential oil of lavender is used in aromatherapy to balance, calm, and soothe on all levels, from burns, scalds, and skin inflammations to nervous tension and insomnia. Lavender essence can help with respiratory problems, sinusitis, headaches, depression, ear infections, urinary tract infections, fevers, shock, and wound-healing. It's a potent natural antibiotic, antiseptic, antispasmodic, antidepressant, and analgesic. Despite its impressive aggressive action against germs and microbes, lavender is one of the only essential oils gentle enough to use undiluted on the skin. However, it works just as well if you dilute it, and given its rarity, expense, and preciousness, it's wise to do so.

Mix ten drops of lavender essence to an ounce of light carrier oil, such as sweet almond or grapeseed. You can carry this in your purse to have on hand for minor emergencies like insect bites, scrapes, and bruises. Sniff lavender essence for stress relief when caught in traffic or dashing about during an overcrowded day.

Definitely keep lavender in the kitchen (next to your aloe vera plant!) as a quick first aid remedy for cuts and scalds. The sooner lavender is applied to a burn or injury, the more effective is its healing power. An excellent treatment for sunburn is to rub the affected skin with fresh aloe vera gel (scraped out from the leaf), then top with a layer of lavender essence mixed with sweet almond oil. This will help take away the redness and discomfort and, depending on the severity of the sunburn, will lessen or eliminate peeling.

Lavender in the bathroom can be used neat (undiluted) in the tub for a relaxing bath and for dabbing onto pimples and skin eruptions. In the bedroom, a nighttime massage with diluted lavender oil helps to promote sleep, as do a few drops of undiluted essence on the pillow. A few drops of the essence can also be added to wash water, the final rinse of your washing machine, or the filter for your dryer to lend a pleasant fragrance and antiseptic boost to domestic cleaning chores.

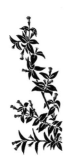

Chapter Three

AROMATHERAPY
FOR WOMEN

Fragrance has been associated with femininity as far back as Isis, the ancient Egyptian goddess. Described five thousand years ago as "The Giver of Life" and "The One Who Is All," her divine aroma was said to nourish and sustain all living things. The Greek goddess Aphrodite, associated with Isis, was guardian of the gods' heavenly perfumes. Paris, who learned some of Aphrodite's aromatic secrets while dallying with one of her handmaidens, created a fragrance so enchanting it wooed Helen away from her husband Menelaus, igniting the Trojan War. Another version of the same story holds that Helen's reputation for great beauty was due not only to her physical attributes but also to an irresistible perfume elixir given her by Aphrodite.

Throughout history women have used fragrance to entice and entrance, to influence and to seduce. When Cleopatra, on her way to meet Antony, sailed up the Nile on her barge, it was so heavily perfumed it could be smelled from miles away. The sails were soaked in floral waters. Aromatic burners wreathed the decks in clouds of fragrance. Bronzed attendants burnished with sweet-smelling oils catered to her as she sat on a dais in a diaphanous gown, the sun's warmth intensifying the aromas of her own potent, custom-blended perfumes. Before business meetings Cleo scented her hair with a heady, intoxicating oil of jasmine. Later, she and Antony made love on a mattress filled with rose petals.

In ancient Egypt, Greece, and Rome, men were just as hedonistic and indulgent in their use of scent as women were, to the point that it became a public nuisance. Julius

Caesar once banned the public use of fragrance, as did Solon of Greece, on grounds that overuse of aromatics was causing allergies among the populace and making it too difficult to breathe. Attempts to legislate the use of perfume may have temporarily cleared the air in the streets, but it could not stamp out its popularity. More than a thousand years after Caesar's ban, in 1760, King George III of England issued an edict that proclaimed that women who seduced men by the use of perfumes could be arrested and imprisoned for the practice of witchcraft.

Fragrance was used as a weapon by the Empress Josephine who, when Napoleon left her, retaliated by having all his rooms soaked in musk, a smell he loathed. Hungary Water, an eau de cologne formulated for the aged queen of Hungary, was said to have transformed a wrinkled old woman into an alluring seductress who soon afterward married the king of Poland. There was even an attempt in 1709 to use perfume as a means of social stratification. A French elitist suggested that a "royal perfume," a "perfume bourgeoisie," and a "perfume for the poor" be formulated to take the guesswork out of class distinction.

As we approach the third millennium, the popularity of fragrance is soaring once again. Precious essences that once were a luxury available only to queens and empresses are relatively easy for us to obtain. For the same amount of money or, in some cases, considerably less than you would spend on an average mass market perfume, you can custom blend a personal fragrance using the finest essences Nature has to offer.

When you go to a department store or boutique to purchase a bottle of perfume, the price tag generally bears little relation to the cost of the ingredients inside the bottle. What you're paying for is packaging and advertising hype—all those billboards, TV commercials, magazine ads, and free samples companies invest millions in to launch a new fragrance. The fragrance itself is a synthetic brew of petrochemicals, or a combination of chemicals and essential oils heavily diluted in water and alcohol. Synthetic aromas are cheaper, easier to standardize, and their smells last longer. However, while certain synthetic fragrances may have psychological associations, they have no physiological or subtle effects and hence they are not used in aromatherapy.

Women and the Sense of Smell

From early childhood on, females are more sensitive to odors and have, on average, a better sense of smell than males. A woman's sense of smell changes during her menstrual cycle, as many aromatherapists, myself included, can tell you. I don't even try to blend during the week of the onset of my period, when my ordinarily acute sense of smell seems almost to turn off. The sense of smell may also become dulled preceding the onset of an illness such as a cold or flu. (If you notice that your nose is less sensitive and it's not related to your usual cycle, reach for preventive essential oils like lavender, eucalyptus, and niaouli and use them with other immunity enhancers such as Vitamin C, zinc, garlic, and echinacea.) Women also tend to alter their odor preferences after the age of forty, which may be related to hormonal changes associated with menopause.

Research indicates that there are very strong links between the sense of smell and sexual function, particularly among females. Aromatherapy educator Michael Scholes suggests that these links may be at the root of our high divorce rates in Western society. By scrubbing off all our natural body odors and then applying synthetic aromas, we present each other with false "smell impressions" and an illusion of compatibility where little or none may actually exist.

Pheromones

Human beings possess more scent glands than any other higher primate. Women have more scent glands than men, concentrated in the armpits and around the nipples, navel, genitalia, and mucous membranes. Among the aromas human beings exude are odorous (though imperceptible on a conscious level) chemicals, known as pheromones, which communicate messages of fear, warning, or sexual attraction. The odors produced by pheromones are not processed through the olfactory system but through a special organ called the VNO, or vomeronasal organ, which looks like a tiny pit just inside of each nostril, barely visible to the naked eye.

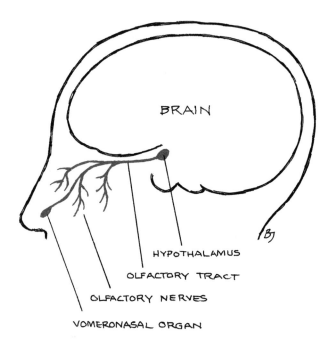

BRAIN

HYPOTHALAMUS

OLFACTORY TRACT

OLFACTORY NERVES

VOMERONASAL ORGAN

Pheromones indicating sexual attraction are emitted by males to affect women, and others given off by women affect men. Pheromones are not aphrodisiacs per se but give the opposite sex a good feeling about us and help to create a relaxed sense of well-being — Nature's way of getting us "in the mood." They may also be used by fetuses to sample the outside world through the amniotic fluid and by infants in the process of learning to recognize their mothers after birth.

Essential oils known as aphrodisiacs may function in much the same way as pheromones by relaxing the body and calming the mind, thereby creating a state in which intimacy is possible. The initial basis of sexual attraction appears to be a largely unconscious process related to the flow of imperceptible chemical messengers between two biologically compatible human beings. The workings of love, however, remain as always a mystery.

Blending

Using and blending essential oils, you can design an entire fragrance "wardrobe" of different blends to fit different moods and purposes. Blends can be formulated purely for the aesthetic pleasure of their aromas. You can also select oils to balance and heal a condition, or to help you in achieving a desired state of mind. When you hit upon a blend that really works for you, you can custom scent all your personal care products to match. Just mix the essential oils separately in a dropper-top glass bottle. Then add a few drops of the premixed blend to unscented shampoos, liquid soaps, shower gels, body oils, and lotions.

The conditions under which you create a blend will influence the quality of the finished product. The same essential oils blended in exactly the same proportions can end up smelling completely different, depending on how, when, and where they were mixed, the ambient temperature, and the level of humidity.

Start with a quiet, fragrance-free room. Silence is best, to allow you to "listen" with your nose to the individual essences as you select them and to the aromatic "music" you create as you blend the oils together. A temperature of 68 to 70 degrees Fahrenheit is ideal.

Set all your materials out before you begin to allow yourself the opportunity to sit quietly and intuitively. It's hard to concentrate if you have to get up every few minutes to find this or that. Have a notebook and a pen handy to record your progress. There's nothing more frustrating than creating the perfect blend, then not being able to remember which oils or how much you used!

When developing a new blend, I generally start with about two ounces of a light-weight carrier oil, such as sweet almond or canola, in a four-ounce bottle. It's easier to mix the essences in an oil, and it's easier to smell how it's coming together as you go along. I find it very difficult to get a true sense of a blend by mixing pure essential oils only, since their concentrated aromas are very intense. Once you've got the proportions for a blend you like, you can mix the essential oils together first without diluting them in a carrier, allowing them time to come together in synergy before adding them to a carrier base.

Blend conservatively! Try starting with three or four pre-chosen essences, adding one or two drops at a time to your carrier and swirling the oil in the bottle gently to mix. Each drop you add will change the character of your blend. To "clear the palate" between intensely aromatic oils, try a sniff of lemon or cedarwood.

The blend is finished when, intuitively, you say "That's just right!" This may not happen every time. That's why I suggest taking your time and going one drop at a time, because making mistakes can be frustrating and expensive. However, like many things in life, the lessons learned from failures are often just as valuable as those learned from success. The more you blend, the better sense you'll develop of which essences blend most effectively, which create the most potent synergies, and which are the fragrances that you like best.

If you are creating a blend for healing purposes, take a few minutes when you're finished to visualize the outcome you'd like to achieve. Hold the oil in your hands, and be specific about what you want it to do. If the blend is for a particular person, create a picture in your mind of that person in a state of radiant health, free of the condition that needs balancing. Your energy and intentions are also ingredients as you create your blend, no less important than the essences chosen and the carrier being used. I also like to take a moment at this point to acknowledge inwardly my appreciation of the earth and the plants, whose life forces I've borrowed to create a healing blend.

Once you have a blend the way you want it, set it aside for a day or two, then smell it again. Depending on the combination of oils you've used, it may change slightly and need some fine tuning. Be aware that when you try to repeat a blend, you may not always get exactly the same results. There can be wide variations in fragrance among essential oils depending on their source. This year's geranium may be very different from last year's and may synergize differently with other oils.

Aromatherapy Perfumes

Once upon a time, perfumes were expected to do much more than just smell pretty. Natural perfume oils and colognes were used to deodorize, disinfect, ward off diseases, and restore lost youth. Napoleon consumed more than 600 bottles per year of the cure-all "aqua mirabilis," or miracle water, an eau de cologne that he sprinkled on himself for personal hygiene, drank as a tonic, and used as an antiseptic to treat wounds on the battlefield. Louis the XIV of France, the "Sun King," had a new mood-altering perfume compounded for him every day of the year.

The art of perfumery is ancient and arcane, with its own culture, customs, and jealously guarded secrets. Borrowing language from the musical realm, perfumers base their approach to blending on the concept of chords. Just as a musical chord is comprised of lower, middle, and top notes, a fragrance chord utilizes essences with different qualities and intensities of fragrance that vibrate harmoniously.

Base notes such as sandalwood, cedar, and spikenard are heavier smelling oils used as fixatives to anchor more fragile and delicate aromas. Animal excretions such as musk, civet, and ambergris have traditionally been used in perfumery as base note fixatives. Middle notes, such as lavender and rosewood, fill up a blend and give it body. Top notes, such as citruses, tend to be lighter, more delicate scents. The top note is what you smell first when you apply a perfume.

Gradually, as the top notes are volatilized into the air by body heat, the middle notes will become apparent, with the base notes lingering longest on the skin.

Aromatherapy perfume oils can be blended in a base of jojoba oil using up to 50 percent essential oil to the carrier base. Be careful with any oils that have the potential for skin irritation, such as spice oils or some of the citruses. Such oils should be used sparingly. If you experience skin irritation from your perfume oil, try diluting it with

Base Notes:

Cistus	Frankincense	Benzoin
Clary Sage	Cedarwood	Oakmoss
Patchouli	Vetiver	Vanilla
Myrrh	Sandalwood	Bay Laurel

Middle Notes:

Rosewood	Marjoram	Palmarosa
Rosemary	Geranium	Spruce
Pine	Tarragon	Lavender
Ginger	Ylang-Ylang	Basil
Chamomile	Nutmeg	Black Pepper

Top Notes:

Bergamot	Lime	Lemongrass
Clove	Anise	Petitgrain
Orange	Peppermint	Balsam Fir
Cardamom	Neroli	Tangerine
Thyme	Angelica	Spearmint
Lemon	Mandarin	Cinnamon
Basil	Juniper berry	

Multi-Note Extenders
(use up to 50 percent to "extend" precious essences)

Jasmine (middle/base)	Lavender	Tangerine
Ylang-Ylang (middle/base)	Rosewood	Palmarosa
Rose (middle/top)	Orange	Geranium (with rose)

Binders
(help to hold a blend together)

Vanilla   Benzoin   Lavender   Rosewood

more carrier oil. If that doesn't solve the problem, discontinue using it and create another blend.

You can also make your own colognes and splashes using an alcohol and water base. Everclear, which is pure grain alcohol, is perfect for this but is not legally available in most states. If you can't get it, try substituting the highest proof vodka you can find. Fill your blending bottle about halfway with the alcohol carrier, add your essential oils, and swirl to mix. When the blend is finished, add more alcohol, leaving room to top off the bottle with about 5 percent distilled water. Give it a gentle shake and put the mixture aside for a month or so, away from sunlight and changing temperatures. Swirl or shake gently about once a week. After the mixture has aged for four to six weeks, strain it through a coffee filter and pour into pretty perfume bottles. You'll want an open top bottle for a splash. Use an atomizer attachment for a spray. A toilet water or splash may use as little as 1 percent to 4 percent essential oil proportionate to the alcohol/water base. A perfume spray can carry an essential oil blend of up to 30 percent. The higher the essential oil content, the more intense and long lasting the scent will be.

Homemade perfume oils and sprays make wonderful gifts, especially when matched with shampoos, shower gels, lotions, and liquid soaps containing the same blends.

Using Essential Oils in the Bath

The easiest way to use essential oils in the bath is simply to drop them in. Because essential oils are lipophilic (attracted to fats) and hydrophobic (they don't diffuse in water) you will see them floating on the surface of the water. Swish your hand through the tub to mix them together, then get in right away, as the steam rising from a warm bath will quickly carry the volatile oils away with it.

Using essential oils neat in the bath can work very well with more dispersible oils such as lavender. But it can be a problem with highly hydrophobic oils such as blue chamomile, which just floats in tight little globs on the water's surface. Using undiluted essences also has the potential to cause irritation, as the concentrated essence comes into direct contact with the skin as you get into the water. This can be a problem for people with extremely sensitive skin.

One way of solving the problem is to premix the hydrophobic or potentially irritating oil with a gentler, more dispersible oil before adding it to the bath. You can also dilute the essences in a bath oil.

Emulsifiers such as milk, egg yolk, or sulfonated castor oil help the essences to disperse uniformly in bath water, but they also cut down on the ability of the essential oil molecules to penetrate the skin. This makes emulsified mixtures less therapeutic but generally doesn't affect the fragrance of the essences.

An aromatic soak in a warm tub of water is a wonderful way to divide a day full of activity from an evening of relaxation and rest. Five to ten drops of pure lavender essence takes all the tension out of a tired body and can help you wind down enough to sleep. A few drops of pure rose essence is the ultimate state-changing bath and is my personal all-time favorite. You can also bathe away many of the symptoms of

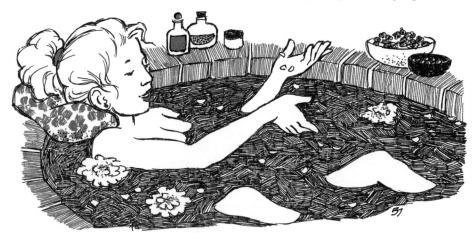

respiratory conditions, urinary tract infections, and skin problems. The antibacterial properties of essential oils help to keep your skin fragrant and healthy. And the antiseptic qualities of the essences make regular aromatic baths an excellent tool in preventing illness from getting hold of you in the first place.

You can use your bathtub as a place of respite, to relax, to rev up for a special evening, or to recover and recuperate, depending on the essences you choose. Try some of the following blends, or make up your own.

Relaxing Baths
5–10 drops lavender, or
2–8 drops rose (geranium or palmarosa are less expensive substitutes), or
2 drops mandarin, 6 drops lavender, 1 drop rosewood, or
2 drops neroli, 4 drops mandarin, or
1 drop marjoram, 2 drops clary sage, 4 drops lavender, 3 drops tangerine.

Stimulating Baths
4 drops rosemary, 6 drops lavender, 1 drop peppermint, or
4–8 drops grapefruit, or
2 drops basil, 4 drops bergamot, or
3 drops lemon, 3 drops thyme linalol, 2 drops eucalyptus, or
2 drops rosemary, 2 drops geranium, 2 drops lavender, 2 drops eucalyptus.

Immune Support Baths
4 drops benzoin, 6 drops lavender, 1 drop each of cypress, rosewood sandalwood, or
3 drops each lavender, tea tree eucalyptus, or
3 drops lemon, 3 drops rosemary, 4 drops lavender, 2 drops thyme, or
3 drops niaouli, 2 drops lemongrass, 4 drops lavender, or
1 drop peppermint, 2 drops orange, 6 drops lavender.

Romantic Baths
2–8 drops rose, or
4–8 drops sandalwood, or
2 drops neroli, 6 drops mandarin (or tangerine), 2 drops sandalwood;
3 drops jasmine, 4 drops bergamot, 2 drops sandalwood, or
3 drops ylang-ylang, 6 drops mandarin, 2 drops cedarwood.

Pre-menstrual syndrome

The bloating, headaches, and mood swings that characterize premenstrual syndrome are caused by the body's response to changing hormonal levels. The process starts

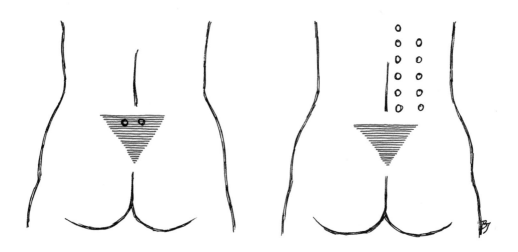

deep within the brain in the hypothalmus, which is, interestingly enough, a part of the limbic system that is directly accessed by essential oils. The hypothalmus influences the pituitary gland, which controls the levels of estrogen and progesterone in the female reproductive system. Changing levels of these hormones result in the ovaries releasing an egg for potential fertilization, which is the point of the whole process.

Stress has an adverse effect on the hypothalmus, which can disrupt the hormonal balance and make PMS worse. Any attempt to alleviate PMS should start with stress reduction. Certain essential oils such as clary sage and fennel have compounds that mimic the molecular structures of female hormones and are popular choices for restoring balance to reproductive processes. Evening primrose and rosa rubignosa oils can have a balancing effect on the female system and can be taken as supplements or added to the carrier base of massage oils. (See "Massage for Women" in the following chapter for massage techniques.)

PMS Baths
2–6 drops rose, or
4 drops lavender, 2 drops clary sage, 1 drop geranium, 2 drops grapefruit, or
3 drops clary sage, 3 drops geranium, 6 drops grapefruit, or
3 drops lemongrass, 2 drops grapefruit, 2 drops geranium, or
2 drops fennel, 4 drops lavender, 1 drop clary sage.

Adieu, Cellulite

Aromatic baths are also an integral part of any genuinely effective cellulite control program. Cellulite is one of those conditions that women believe in and most men don't because they're not prone to it. I know many doctors who have proclaimed that only one kind of fat is produced by the human body. I have heard a male aromatherapist say that cellulite will disappear of its own accord with an active sex life. (It does not!) Men may be able to stand naked in front of a full-length mirror and say, "There's no such thing as cellulite," but for women it's not that easy, especially if we have to turn around!

Maurice Messegue, the famous French herbalist who treated Winston Churchill, King Farouk, and Jean Cocteau, among many others, is the only male practitioner I'm aware of who has taken cellulite as seriously as women do. He viewed cellulite as a condition symptomatic of a clogged and sluggish system, the result of an over-processed, pesticide-contaminated daily diet and sedentary lifestyle. He links it to a precancerous condition.

Whether or not you're ready to take cellulite that seriously, the good news is that you can do something about it. Aromatic baths and oils help to drain excess fluids and tone, stimulate, and strengthen the entire system while improving the appearance, texture, and elasticity of the skin. Essences such as benzoin, birch, clary sage, cypress, cedar, eucalyptus, fennel, geranium, grapefruit, helichrysum, juniper, lemon, lemongrass, peppermint, pine, rosemary, tea tree, and thyme can be used singly or in combination. However, essential oils can only do so much. Dietary changes and plenty of exercise are an absolute must.

Integral to cellulite control is daily dry brushing of the skin with a natural bristle brush. Dry brushing removes dead cells from the skin's surface and helps to stimulate the lymphatic system. Body brushes come with bristles that have varying degrees of stiffness, and you'll need to test different brushes against your skin to find the one that's right for you. What you want is one that's stiff enough to stimulate and exfoliate your skin without tearing it or causing undue discomfort. Make sure you get a brush with natural bristles. (It usually says so on the handle.) Plastic bristles can damage the skin.

Dry brush your skin *every day*, starting with the bottoms of the feet, brushing in upward strokes toward the heart. You can sprinkle a few drops of a good draining, detoxifying oil such as cypress, juniper, or lemon onto the bristles for added effect. The whole process only takes a minute or two, and the results are well worth your time. You'll brush your feet, legs, thighs, buttocks, belly, arms, and back. Don't try to brush your chest, breasts, neck, or face. The skin there is too delicate and you may end up with broken capillaries and sore spots. A good thorough body brushing before your morning shower can be very stimulating as you start the day. You may also want to brush before an evening bath to polish your skin silky smooth in preparation for a special night.

Dr. Valnet suggests a blend of fresh chamomile and lemon to prevent weight gain. Take two heads of chamomile and a sliced lemon, pour a cup of boiling water over them, and leave it to sit overnight. In the morning, strain and drink before eating breakfast.

Seaweed is another good toner and detoxifier. Try throwing a handful of powdered kelp (available at health food stores) into a warm bath before you add your essential oils. It's messy, but it helps.

After your bath or shower, you'll want to do a quick all-over body massage with a cellulite-fighting blend of essential oils in a skin-nourishing nut oil base. Try some of my suggestions, or create your own formulations.

Cellulite Control Baths
6 drops grapefruit, 3 drops cypress, 1 drop rosemary, 1 drop thyme, or
2 drops lemon, 2 drops cypress, 2 drops fennel, 2 drops benzoin, or
1 drop birch, 2 drops lemongrass, 2 drops geranium, or
2 drops cedarwood, 2 drops juniper, 1 drop clary sage, 1 drop rosemary, or
3 drops eucalyptus, 2 drops pine, 1 drop rosemary, 1 drop peppermint.

Skin Care with Essential Oils

While there are a number of "aromatherapy" skin care lines that use essential oils in their formulations, in my experience most of these products tend to be very expensive and not always effective. To prolong shelf life and to be safe for public consumption, mass-marketed products are required to contain preservatives as well. Many so-called natural skin care products contain substantial amounts of standard cosmetic ingredients that don't do much of anything for anybody beyond filling up the bottle or jar.

I'm talking about mineral oils, waxes, and synthetic chemical compounds that are at best inert and at worst cause allergic reactions in sensitive skin.

It's so easy to make your own skin care cosmetics! If you can cook, you can make creams, soaps, and cleansers in less time and with considerably less effort than it takes to make breakfast or lunch, and there's less washing up afterward too.

All you need is a double boiler or bain marie, a blender or food processor, a wire whisk or beater, a few ingredients, a sense of adventure, and a little time. Most of the ingredients can be purchased at a health food or herb store (or check the "Resource Guide" at the end of the book). Without preservatives your cosmetics will last for several weeks, depending on the ingredients you use and whether or not you refrigerate them. Adding essential oils will have some antibacterial effect on your preparations, but won't make them last forever. I think that's a good thing. Cosmetics should ultimately be food for the skin, and in most cases fresh food is better. With the money you save making your own skin care products, you can buy some wonderful essences to work with—quality essences of rose, neroli, and jasmine that are simply too expensive for large manufacturers to use in more than trace amounts. Of course, you don't have to use precious oils to create effective skin care products. There are plenty of less expensive alternatives for every skin type.

Following are some suggestions for skin care products that are similar to what you might be using or have used in the past. They break down into three basic steps— cleansing, toning, and moisturizing. Feel free to experiment! Once you have the basics down, you can create your own variations.

Essential Oils for Oily Skin: Cypress, eucalyptus, geranium, lavender, niaouli, palmarosa, rosewood.

Essential Oils for Acne and Pimples: Bergamot, carrot seed, cedarwood, geranium, lavender, myrrh, orange, palmarosa, rosemary, rosewood, sandalwood. (Lavender and rosewood can be dabbed onto pimples. The other oils should be diluted in a cleanser, toner or moisturizer before being applied to the skin.)

Essential oils for normal or combination skin: Carrot seed, clary sage, geranium, lavender, palmarosa, rosewood.

Essential Oils for Dry Skin: Benzoin, carrot seed, geranium, lavender, neroli, palmarosa, rose, rosemary, rosewood, sandalwood.

Essential Oils for Sensitive Skin: Carrot seed, jasmine, lavender, marjoram, neroli, rose, rosewood.

Essential Oils for Couperose Skin (broken capillaries): Cypress, helichrysum, lavender, rosewood, sandalwood.

CLEANSERS

The purpose of a cleanser is simply to remove dirt and excess oil from the surface of the skin. Many commercially available soaps are based on harsh defatting detergents. That "squeaky clean" feeling means your skin has been stripped of all the natural oils that normally protect and moisturize it.

Still, there are many women who don't feel their skin is truly clean if they haven't used soap. Essential oils can be added to a store-bought, unscented liquid facial soap, or try the following.

Liquid Soap Cleanser for Oily or Normal Skin

Grate a bar of a gentle, vegetable-based unscented soap into a pot, and add it to a quart of bottled water. Heat the mixture on the stove, stirring until the grated soap is completely dissolved. This is your liquid soap base. When the mixture has cooled, take out about eight ounces of it and mix in 8–10 drops of essential oil: lavender, rosemary, lemon, geranium, thyme, linalol, and rosewood are all good choices, either singly or in combination. Put the scented soap into a bottle or pump-top container. The remainder can be put aside in a larger bottle or jar to refill your daily use bottle as necessary. Use the soap sparingly, diluting it further in your hands with water when you wash, and rinse well. To give the liquid soap a "scrubbing" action, add a tablespoon of ground almond before you add the essential oils (you can grind the nuts in your blender, food processor, or coffee bean grinder) and mix thoroughly. Shake well before each use.

Chamomile Milk Cleanser for Dry or Sensitive Skin

Put a cup of half-and-half or creamy milk into a bain marie or double boiler. Add half a cup of fresh or dried chamomile flowers, and heat for half an hour just below the boiling point, stirring frequently. Take it off the heat and let sit for a couple of hours, then strain the liquid into a bottle or jar. Add a few drops of lavender, blue chamomile, or helichrysum essential oil and stir well, then refrigerate. When you get up in the morning, take out just what you'll need for the day and let it warm to near room temperature before using it with a cotton ball on your face. Rinse with tepid water, or wipe with a soft cloth or tissue.

Scrubby Almond Cleansing Paste for Oily, Normal or Dry Skin

This is a variation on a cleansing paste recipe included in Valerie Worwood's excellent book *The Fragrant Pharmacy*. Grind almonds until you have about half a cup of them, then throw them in a blender (if they're not there already) with one-fourth cup of sweet almond oil, two tablespoons of apple cider vinegar, and two tablespoons of water (bottled or floral). Add six drops of the essential oil of your choice and blend until it makes a smooth paste. (Try lemon, lavender, or thyme linalol for oily skin; lavender, geranium, clary sage, or rosewood for normal skin; helichrysum or blue chamomile for sensitive or couperose skin; lavender, sandalwood, or a couple drops of rose, jasmine, or neroli for dry skin.) This mixture separates when it sits around and will need to be stirred each time you use it. Remove what you need with a spoon to avoid introducing bacteria from your hands. This is a really nice cleanser and will leave your skin clear, moist, and radiant. Rub a small amount gently into the skin and rinse well with tepid water.

Two-Thousand-Year-Old Cold Cream

This recipe is adapted from a cold cream recipe recorded by the ancient Greek physician Galen. The original was called Ceratum Galeni, Galen's Cold Cream. In a bain marie or double boiler put an ounce of beeswax and an ounce of boric acid (Galen used spermaceti), adding 16 ounces of sweet almond oil. Heat and stir until everything is liquefied. Remove from heat and, while beating constantly, dribble in 16 ounces of rose water (the floral water should be room temperature or warmer). When the mixture has cooled down, add eight to ten drops of rose attar (otto, or absolute; geranium or palmarosa will also do). Spoon into jars, and use as a cleansing cream and makeup remover.

TONERS

Toners remove any cleanser residue from the skin, tighten the pores, and improve overall texture. In my opinion, aromatic floral waters—by-products of the essential oil distillation process—make the best toners. They can be misted on from spray bottles or applied with cotton balls. To make them more economical, they can also be diluted up to 50 percent with witch hazel. For dry or sensitive skin, add a couple drops of liquid glycerine to the floral water/witch hazel mixture and shake well before each use.

The best-quality floral waters come from the same places you would find quality essential oils and herbal products. Lesser-quality rose and orange blossom floral waters can generally be found in pharmacies and liquor stores and at Middle Eastern specialty stores. Floral waters are perishable and should be kept refrigerated when not being used.

MOISTURIZERS

A good moisturizer should do more than just make the surface of the skin slick and slippery. The ingredients should be able to penetrate down into the deeper layers to support skin functions and rejuvenate newly forming skin cells. Essential oils are perfectly suited for this, especially when used in conjunction with other skin-nourishing ingredients.

Rose hip seed oil, *Rosa rubignosa* or *R. mosqueta,* makes an excellent carrier base for an essential oil blend suited to your skin type. This oil supports skin metabolism and regenerative processes through its high content of essential fatty acids; it also supports underlying physiological functions. You can use it alone or in combination with other oils such as hazelnut or jojoba (a few drops of this will do). Add a few drops of carrot seed oil for extra skin support, and a Vitamin E capsule, or a few drops of wheat germ oil to preserve your blend and keep it from becoming rancid. Facial oils should be mixed in small quantities— an ounce or less at a time. You will probably want to apply a facial oil several times a day for best results.

Here is a recipe for a good, light moisturizing cream that can be used on the face or the body. It's absorbed into the skin quickly and easily. The cocoa butter has a fairly strong chocolaty smell, so it's good to use intensely aromatic essential oils such as citruses, clary sage, geranium, or ylang-ylang to balance it.

All-Over Moisturizing Cream

1 ounce cocoa butter
1 ounce shea butter
8 ounces sweet almond, sesame, or hazelnut oil
6 ounces floral water
4–8 drops essential oils

In a bain marie or double boiler, melt the cocoa butter and shea butter with the oil. Remove from the heat source and add room temperature (or slightly warmed) floral water, beating or stirring constantly until cool. (Don't stop or the mixture will separate!) Add the essential oils to the cooled creamy mixture. It will seem a little thin and may separate a bit at the top after you pour it into bottles. Just give it a good shake before you use it. Because of the cocoa butter, the moisturizer will seem to be thin for a few days, then it will thicken slightly to a creamier texture.

Facial Steams and Packs

Another good way to get essential oils into the skin is with steam. All you need is a bowl or basin of hot water, a towel, and the essential oils of your choice. Let the water cool slightly from boiling so the steam doesn't scald you and the essences don't evaporate too quickly. Put 8–10 drops of essential oil into the hot water, tent a towel over your head, and let the steam penetrate your skin. You can also use a combination of fresh herbs and essential oils in the same way.

Add essential oils to your cleansing and purifying facial masks as well. Powdered clays are available at health food stores and bath and body boutiques and can be used on face and body to give skin a deep cleansing and nourishing lift. Mix with floral water and add essential oils. For dry skin, you can also add honey or glycerine for a moisturizing dimension.

Try a mask of egg white with two teaspoons of honey with essential oils for oily skin.

Ripe avocado makes an excellent facial pack for dry skin, mixed with a little yogurt and a spoonful of honey, along with essential oils for dry skin. Even simpler is a rehydrating mask of mashed ripe bananas, with sandalwood. To calm irritated skin, blend grapes with a spoonful of honey and several drops of lavender. To smoothe out expression lines, try a mask of two egg yolks, two teaspoons of avocado or hazelnut oil, oatmeal to thicken, a little lemon juice, and three drops of neroli.

Here's a recipe for an all-over moisturizing pack. This is a heavy cream. Rub it into the skin of your face and body before getting into the shower, then scrub well with a loofah under warm water. It's a quick treatment to leave your whole body feeling polished and silky smooth.

All-Over Moisturizing Pack
8 ounces avocado, hazelnut, or wheat germ oil
6 ounces floral water
1 ounce beeswax
Several drops of essential oil of your choice

In a bain marie or double boiler, melt the oil and wax together. Remove from heat and whip in the floral water (room temperature or warmed), stirring or beating continuously until cooled. Then stir in the essential oils and pour into widemouth jars. This cream thickens as it cools and will probably have to be removed from the jar with a spoon.

Carrier Oils

Essential oils can be mixed into any unscented cream, shampoo, lotion, or oil. That which the essence is mixed into is called a "carrier," since it "carries" the essential oil into contact with the skin. In addition, the following base oils provide nourishment to the skin with vitamins, minerals, and proteins. For massage and skin care, use only cold-pressed oils free of solvent residue.

Sweet Almond Oil: A stable oil, highly nutritious, and easily absorbed into the skin. One of the best all-round choices for massage and skin care. Good oil to use on children.

Apricot Kernel Oil: Another nourishing oil, not as stable as sweet almond.

Avocado Oil: Very rich, heavy oil especially good for dry, sunburned, or dehydrated skin. Combine with lighter oil to speed absorption.

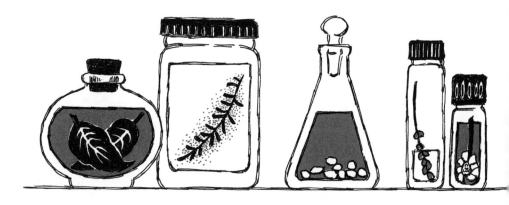

Canola Oil: Good basic massage oil, stable due to high linoleic acid content. Pressed from rapeseed. Light and quick to absorb.

Corn Oil: Easy to find, nourishing, but not very stable — goes rancid quickly.

Grapeseed Oil: Very light, quick to absorb.

Hazelnut Oil: Rich, nourishing, gives smooth texture to skin.

Olive Oil: Good for hair care and in combination with other oils. Tends to be a bit too sticky and strong smelling to use alone.

Peanut Oil: Good basic massage oil, easy to find.

Safflower Oil: Good basic massage oil, suitable for all skin types.

Sesame Oil: Light and nourishing, especially recommended for children in the Indian medical practice of Ayurveda for its warming quality. Virgin cold-pressed oil contains natural antioxidants, which increase its stability. Refined sesame oil is better for

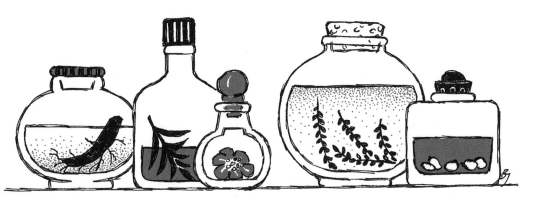

aromatherapy purposes—unrefined oil has a strong "food" smell that overpowers the essences.

Sunflower Oil: Good basic massage oil.

Specialty Oils

These oils, added to the base oils listed above, boost their healing and nourishing power.

Use up to 10 percent in your carrier oil base. These fragile oils should be kept in the refrigerator. They tend to go rancid quickly when exposed to heat or sunlight.

Borage Seed Oil: Contains vitamins, minerals, and is comprised of up to one-fourth gamma linoleic acid (GLA). GLA reinforces the ability of the skin to function as a protective membrane. Healing and regenerating to skin. Use in facial oils and for psoriasis, eczema, and aging skin. Also supports underlying physiological functions of the cardiovascular system and is a good oil to use for women who suffer from PMS or menopause-related ups and downs. Used in Europe to treat multiple sclerosis.

Carrot Seed Oil: Actually an essential oil. Contains vitamins, minerals, and beta carotene. Rejuvenating, good for all skin problems.

Evening Primrose Oil: Another GLA-rich oil, also useful for balancing PMS and other female hormone-related problems. Used in Europe to treat hyperactivity in children, hypertension, to reduce cholesterol levels and soothe skin irritations. Also used to treat multiple sclerosis.

Jojoba Oil: Not an oil but a wax. Doesn't go rancid. Perfect base for perfume oils. Good hair conditioning oil. A few drops can be added to facial oils to increase emollience.

Rosehip Seed Oil: (*Rosa mosqueta, Rosa rubignosa*) Also rich in GLA. Properties similar to evening primrose. Another excellent oil for face and skin care, nutritious to the skin, emollient and regenerative.

Wheat Germ Oil: Very rich, with high content of vitamins E, A, and B. Good antioxidant. Useful for all skin conditions. Use up to 10 percent in a blend with other carrier oils to increase emollience and retard spoilage.

Diffusors

One of the easiest ways to use essential oils for aromatherapy is in a diffusor. The most therapeutically effective diffusors are those that "nebulize" the essential oil into a thin mist by forcing air through the essence and spraying it into the air. These diffusors generally come equipped with a small motor, like the one that would blow air into your aquarium, and a glass chimney that screws onto the top of a bottle or vial of essential oil. Diffusors can be run for one to five minutes every one to three hours for children, and up to ten minutes an hour for adults.

A simple, low-tech diffusor design is very similar to a potpourri burner. A small cup rests a few inches atop a heat source, such as a candle or light bulb. The essential oils can be floated on top of a bit of water in the diffusor cup and evaporate as the water heats up. Some of these, designed in glass, ceramic, or porcelain, can be really beautiful.

Ceramic light bulb rings can be used for the same purpose and are much less expensive. However, their drawback is that the heat from the light bulb may cause the essences to volatilize too rapidly. The heat may also cause chemical changes in the oil itself, affecting the therapeutic abilities of the oil.

Most steam vaporizers come equipped with a small well for medicaments. This is a perfect place to put in a few drops of a respiratory or preventive blend, such as lavender, tea tree, and eucalyptus.

The simplest diffusor is a bowl of hot water placed on a table or radiator, with a few drops of essential oil added. Try creating your own blends using the following suggestions:

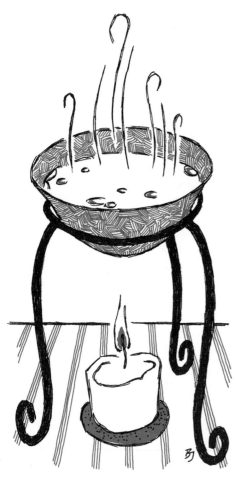

Relaxing Oils: Lavender, geranium, chamomile, clary sage, marjoram, eucalyptus, jasmine, rose, ylang-ylang, mandarin, neroli.

Stimulating Oils: Rosemary, peppermint, basil, bergamot, grapefruit.

Uplifting Oils: Tangerine, orange, cedarwood, lemon, pine, rosewood, frankincense.

Respiratory Oils: Eucalyptus, pine, niaouli, tea tree, ravensara, lemon, rosemary, peppermint.

Aphrodisiac Oils: Jasmine, rose, sandalwood, cedarwood, neroli, clary sage, ylang-ylang.

Dilutions: When diluting essential oils in a carrier, use a 2–3 percent essence to carrier ratio for adults; 1–1.5 percent ratio for children over the age of two; .5 percent or less for children under the age of two; and even less for babies. To be perfectly accurate it's best to work by weight using a scale that measures in milligrams. The amount of essential oil contained in a "drop" can vary greatly depending on the size of the dropper opening and the viscosity of the essence being dispensed. The following recommendations are approximate for this reason.

Bath

Adults: 5–15 drops, depending on the essences used

Children: 3–5 drops of child safe essences (see page 84 for list).

Babies: 1–2 drops of extremely gentle essences such as rose, lavender, or chamomile.

Massage
Adults: Up to 15 drops per ounce of carrier.
Children: Up to 8 drops per ounce of carrier.
Babies: 1–2 drops per ounce of carrier.

Perfume
Adults: Up to 50 percent essential oil to a jojoba oil base, depending on essences used
Children: Up to 20 percent essential oil to jojoba oil base, child-safe oils only.
Babies: Do not use perfumes or colognes on babies.
Conversions: Essential oils are usually sold by metric weight or volume. Following are some approximate conversions between various measurements you may encounter:

> 20 drops = 1 ml essential oil
> 5 ml = 1 teaspoon
> 15 ml = 1 tablespoon
> 300 drops = 15 ml essential oil
> 15 ml = half an ounce
> 30 ml = 1 ounce
> 1 fluid dram = 3.697 ml
> 1 tsp. = 1.3 fl. drams
> 8 fl. drams = 1 fl. ounce
> 16 drams = 1 ounce (weight)
> 1 dram = 1.772 grams

Aromatic Gardening

The best way to get to know essential oils really intimately is to grow the plants that produce them and distill them yourself. A primitive distillation setup can be created in your kitchen using a teapot with a spout, a plastic hose, a bowl of ice, and a container to collect the distilled product. Fill the teapot with the fresh plant material you want to distill. Attach a plastic hose to the spout, where the steam comes out. Run the hose through a bowl or bucket of ice, to cool the steam, then let the end drip down into another container to collect the condensation. The essential oil will float on top and can be taken off with patient use of a glass eye dropper with a rubber squeeze bulb. The distilled water that is left over can be used for soaps, lotions, or skin care.

Of course, it's not possible to use this method with every oil. Plants that produce essential oils come from all over the world, and some won't grow anywhere other than their native soil. However, there are some herbs and flowers that can be grown almost anywhere, at least seasonally, and I encourage you to make their acquaintance. Herbs such as rosemary and thyme can be planted outside or in a kitchen window garden, then used in cooking and for cosmetics and medicinals. Flowers such as rose and jasmine add grace to any home through the beauty of their blossoms and fragrance, as their essences are released naturally into the air.

Here are some aromatic plants for you to try in your own garden. I've preselected plants that produce essential oils and are historically useful and easy to grow. Take time to get to know them, as you would new friends, and I can promise that your affection and attention to them will be amply repaid.

BASIL Ocimum basilicum

*The smell of Basil is good for the heart. It taketh away
sorrowfulness, which commeth of melancholy and maketh a
man merry and glad.*

FROM *Gerard's Herbal*, 1597

This is one of my all-time favorite herbs. It's a prolific,
easy-to-grow annual that likes a sunny, well-drained
location. Cut it back frequently to keep it bushy, giving
it a little fertilizer afterward.

In India, a variety of basil known as tulasi is a
sacred plant, second only to the lotus, and grows near
every temple and home as a protective talisman. Oaths
are sworn in court with basil, which is consecrated to
the Hindu gods Vishnu and Krishna. Its stems are used
as rosaries, and the herb is believed to open the heart
and mind and to strengthen faith, compassion, and clarity. Hindu dead are washed with basil water and carry a
leaf of it with them into the afterlife. In Persia, Egypt,
and Malaysia, basil is planted on graves. In Haiti, basil
is sacred to the love goddess Erzulie, and its use brings
her divine protection. In Mexico, basil is carried in the
pockets to attract money and love. In Italy, women put
a pot of basil in the window to let a lover know he is
expected. Arabs use it to combat drunkenness, and in
South America it is used to bring visionary natives out
of shamanic trance states. Basil was found to be growing around Christ's tomb after the resurrection, and in
the Greek Orthodox church it is still used to prepare
holy water. The French have a saying, "semer le

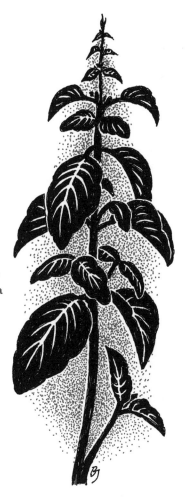

basilic," which means to hurl abuse, derived from an ancient Greek and Roman idea that basil must be cursed as it is sown to ensure germination. (Let me know if this works. I have neighbors living too close by to try it myself!)

Basil is said to absorb positive ions, energize negative ions, and liberate beneficial ozone. In cooking, it goes really well with tomatoes. Try adding a few fresh leaves to tomato sauce or soup, along with thyme and bay laurel. It's also delicious in omelets and scrambled eggs. The fresh leaves can be preserved in oil or vinegar—just make sure they're completely dry before you put them in the bottle.

Purple basil makes a beautiful ruby red-colored vinegar. Fill a bottle about a third of the way with fresh herb, adding some regular basil leaves for flavor, and let it sit in the sun for a week, bringing it in at night. Then remove most of the plant matter from the bottle to show off the color. It makes a wonderful salad dressing. You can also chop or process fresh basil with garlic, olive oil, pine nuts, and parmesan cheese to make your own pesto. This freezes nicely and lets you bring some of your summer garden in to brighten up winter menus.

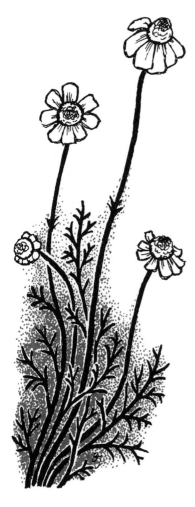

CHAMOMILE Anthemis nobilis, Matricaria chamomilla

For though the chamomile, the more it is trodden on the faster it grows, yet youth, the more it is wasted, the sooner it wears.

FALSTAFF, IN SHAKESPEARE'S *Henry IV*

Chamomile gets its name from the Greek *khamaimelon*, meaning "ground apple," perhaps because since the time of the ancient temple of Thessaly the herb has been planted as a ground cover and has been trodden on, releasing its sweet, fruity fragrance. It was the favorite herb of the Egyptians, who dedicated it to the sun and revered its healing properties and used it to reduce fevers and ease rheumatism. Greek physicians prescribed chamomile for female disorders. The Romans believed it was an antidote to snakebite. Chamomile has been used medicinally in many parts of the world, from Europe to Russia, where it is known as *romashka*, India, where it's called *babunah*, and Mexico and South America, where it has taken the Spanish name *manzanilla*, which translates as "little apple of the earth," an interesting similarity to the Greek.

Under its old Saxon name *maythen*, chamomile was one of the nine sacred herbs believed to be effective against the "flying venoms" carried by the wind and blamed by ancient Europeans as the cause of diseases. It has been used since pre-Christian times to treat eye inflammations. An old gardening tradition claims that chamomile scattered about the garden will keep all the plants healthy.

If you have the time and patience to pick enough of those teeny tiny little flowers to make a pot of tea, it's a wonderful nightcap to bring on sweet dreams. (Or try mixing just a few chamomile flowers in with easier to pick leaves of another soothing herb, such as melissa or marjoram.) Chamomile tea is also a good tummy soother and digestive aid. An infusion of chamomile, fresh or dried, can be used as a rinse after shampooing to brighten blond hair, and according to Mexican tradition, bathing in the flowers makes the body more beautiful.

An infusion or tea of chamomile is also a great pick-me-up for tired eyes, and I've found the floral water to be very effective in compresses to ease the irritation caused by conjunctivitis. Simply soak a cotton ball and put it over the closed eye, then lie down for fifteen minutes or so. Keep the infused tea or floral water refrigerated and take it out a few minutes before using to let it warm just slightly. The chill of refrigeration can be a bit intense for sensitive eyes.

FENNEL Foeniculum vulgare

Seeds, leaves and root of our garden Fennel are much used in drinks and broths for those that are grown fat, to abate their unwieldiness and cause them to grow more gaunt and lank.

WILLIAM COLES (ELIZABETHAN), 1650

The ancient Greek word for fennel was *marathron*, from *maraino*, meaning "to grow thin." During the Middle Ages, it was used as an appetite suppressant during Lent and fast days.

There's something magical about this easy-to-grow herb, especially when it reaches its full height of six or seven feet. A garden with a corner full of feathery, licorice-scented leaves gives children the feeling of being in a fairy forest. Fennel is a perennial plant in milder climates, though it's usually grown as a summer annual. It likes light, well-drained soil and lots of sun and is very drought-tolerant.

Back in Roman times, branches of fennel were used to beat disobedient students. Pliny recommended fennel for twenty-two different ailments. His recommendations led to traditional beliefs that the juice of fennel sharpened the sight. Fennel roots boiled in wine were applied to the eyes to cure cataracts. Fennel is another of the nine sacred healing herbs mentioned in the ancient Saxon *Lacnunga*. It was used for protection against witchcraft and the evil eye and as an antidote to snakebites and venom. The herb was brought to North America by the Spaniards and still grows wild around some of the old missions. English herbalist Nicholas Culpeper suggested drinking an infusion of the seeds boiled in water to relieve hiccups, ease stomach cramps, and stop gas pains. Boiling the seeds in wine made an antidote to toxic plants and mushrooms. The crushed seeds made an expectorant tea. Native Americans boiled fennel seeds and leaves in barley water to increase the quality and amount of milk produced by a nursing mother.

You can use fennel stalks and leaves as a garnish for fish and in salads, or try herb enthusiast Patrick Lima's calming digestive-aid tea, which combines fresh sweet fennel with lemon balm (melissa) and spearmint leaves. Fennel gives an aromatic kick to vegetables, spaghetti sauce, and chicken. Leave the seeds to ripen if you want to attract wild birds to your garden, or harvest them before they fall and use them to season breads and puddings, or chew as a digestive aid.

JASMINE Jasminum officinale

This is a wonderful flowering shrub to plant outside windows that will be left open in summer. There are many varieties of jasmine from which to choose. The *Jasminum officinale grandiflorum*, or "Spanish jasmine" from which the absolute is derived, is a semievergreen to deciduous vine that blooms all summer. *Jasminum officinale*, the "common white" or "poet's jasmine," is similar to the *grandiflorum* but has smaller flowers and requires a milder climate. *Jasminum sambac*, or "Arabian jasmine," is the evergreen shrub known in Hawaii as *pikake*, used in leis and perfumes. It is also used in the Orient to make jasmine tea.

MARJORAM Origanum majorana

Like basil, this is a good plant to grow outside in a garden, or in windowsill containers indoors. Marjoram likes the sun and good drainage. Make sure you keep it well trimmed and cut off the blossoms when they appear to sustain the plant's growth. In milder climates, marjoram is a perennial; in colder zones, an annual.

Gerard, in his sixteenth-century herbal, suggests marjoram for those "who are given to over-much sighing." The Greeks, who called it "joy of the mountains," believed that its scent was created by Aphrodite as a symbol of happiness. Bridal couples were crowned with garlands of marjoram, and the plants were placed on graves to give peace to departed spirits. Romans offered bunches of marjoram as symbols of peace and friendship.

Grown in the garden, it attracts butterflies and bees. A tea of fresh marjoram leaves with honey promotes sleep and soothes sore throats and colds. It's a popular remedy among singers to preserve the voice. The fresh leaves can also be chopped fine and added to salads and fish, or in the last minutes of cooking to meat dishes. Traditionally, marjoram has been used as an antidote to narcotic poisons and convulsions and in a warm infusion at the onset of measles to cause sweating and bring out the skin eruptions.

PEPPERMINT Mentha piperita

Grow mint in your garden to attract money to your purse.

EUROPEAN SAYING

There are many varieties of mint, and these hardy perennials will quickly take over your garden if you give them any encouragement, such as plenty of water and partial shade. A variation, *Mentha piperita citrata*, orange or bergamot mint, produces an aromatic leaf that has a slight orange flavor when crushed. *Mentha spicata*, or spearmint, has smaller leaves, a milder flavor, and less stimulating effect.

Mint played an important part in the ancient Greek mysteries and was believed to have the power to reanimate spirits. According to Greek mythology, Pluto turned his mistress into a mint plant to protect her from his jealous wife. Peppermint was used medicinally by the Egyptians and was prescribed by Hippocrates as a stimulant and diuretic. Roman women, for whom drinking wine was a capital offense, used mint to mask any odor of alcohol on the breath.

Traditionally, mint was believed to prevent milk from curdling and, when combined with salt, to be effective against the bite of mad dogs. In ancient Israel, the Pharisees collected tithes in mint, and the Hebrews laid it on the temple floor. It was later used in Italian churches, where it was sacred to the Madonna and went by the name "Erba Santa Maria." Mint is also used medicinally in Mexico and South America, where it is known as *yerba buena*.

John Parkinson, who served as apothecary to King James I, noted in his seventeenth-century herbal, "Mints are sometimes used in the bath with balm and other herbs to comfort and strengthen the nerves and sinews." The bruised leaves were bound on the forehead to relieve headaches.

Mint leaves are most aromatic just before the plant flowers. The leaves can be used in teas or salads and are useful for tummy troubles and digestive upsets. Peppermint tea can be very stimulating and makes a good substitute for coffee.

ROSE Rosa centifolia, R. damascena, R. gallica, etc.

"Among all floures of the worlde the floure of the rose is cheyf and beeryth ye pryse."
FROM *Bartholomew's Herbal*, THIRTEENTH CENTURY

Four thousand years ago, an artisan carved the image of a rose into the walls of the Palace of Knossos in Crete. Egyptians loved roses as well and exported them to Rome, where the hedonistic Romans ran rose water through their fountains and bathed in rose wine. The petals were used in cosmetics and dried and powdered for use after the bath as an antiperspirant.

To the Greeks, the rose was a symbol of love, beauty, and happiness and got its red color from Aphrodite's blood. The Thracian King Midas, known to us as the man whose touch turned everything to gold, was better known in his own time for his finely scented rose garden.

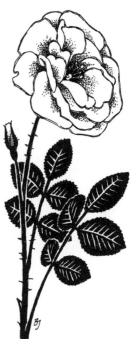

Roses were used in alchemy, and Avicenna, the great Arab physician of the tenth century, is credited as being the first to have distilled the essence. A Persian princess who had her fountains filled with rose water on her wedding day detected the essence floating on top and named it Attar, after her husband. In Arabic Spain, the clothing of the emirs was rinsed in rose water. Muslims claimed that the rose sprang from the sweat of Mohammad's brow and conscripted Bulgarian peasants to cultivate it. The Bulgarian rose, originally imported from Damascus, Syria, by the Ottoman Turks, is botanically identical to wild roses growing in the foothills of the Himalayas.

The fragrance of roses, especially of the "old roses" that have not been hybridized, makes them pure joy to bring indoors to perfume the house. A gardening tradition says that parsley, grown near rosebushes, will enhance their aroma. Rose petals can be dried for potpourri or used fresh to make rosewater, medicinal conserves, and honey. The sixteenth century *Ashkam's Herbal* gives a recipe for "Melrosette" in which fresh red rose petals, with the white heel removed, are chopped up small and boiled in purified honey. "To know when it is boyled ynoughe, ye shall know it by the swete odour and the colour read." Ashkam claimed this honey would keep for five years and possessed the "vertues" of cleansing the system and comforting the heart.

ROSEMARY Rosmarinus officinalis

Where Rosemary flourishes, the lady rules.
Europeean saying

Smell it oft and it shall keep thee youngly.
From *Banckes' Herbal*, sixteenth century

Its name is derived from the Latin *ros marinus*, or "dew of the sea." Rosemary was sacred to the Romans, was burned as an incense in ancient Greece, and has been found in Egyptian tombs. Greek students tucked a bit of the herb over their ears before examinations to sharpen the mind. Ancient hunters stuffed game with rosemary to prevent the meat from rotting, and it remains a popular culinary herb. In the Middle Ages, rosemary was used in exorcisms to drive out evil spirits and was widely believed to bring good luck and to prevent the effects of witchcraft. It was also used as a symbol of faithfulness. Branches of rosemary were strewn in courts to prevent the spread of typhus, or "jail fever," and it was burned with juniper berries in French hospitals to deodorize and disinfect.

In mild climates rosemary is a perennial and can grow into a shrub that is practically the size of a tree. In fact its wood was once used to make boxes, lutes, and carpenter's rules. It's a good plant to grow in a container if you don't have room for a garden. Keep it near the kitchen so you can pinch off the aromatic leaves as necessary for cooking. Stalks of fresh or dried rosemary can be put in among linens to give them a warm, herbal fragrance and to repel moths and other insects. Or make a rosemary-flavored cooking and salad oil by filling a jar with the fresh herb (make sure it's dry) and setting it in a sunny kitchen window for a couple of weeks. Remove the herb and strain.

Banckes' Herbal is full of suggestions for using rosemary, such as putting a sprig under your pillow to chase away bad dreams. He also suggests putting rosemary leaves among clothes and books. A beauty tip: "Boyle the leaves in white wine and washe thy face therewith and thy browes and thou shalt have a faire face." "Also, if thou be feeble boyle the leaves in cleane water and washe thyself and thou shalt wax shiny." The same "boyled" rosemary water, mixed with an equal amount of white wine, was used in soups to restore the appetite. Rosemary stalks can be burned, according to Banckes, and the powder rubbed on the teeth to keep them strong and healthy. Rosemary is also good "for ye weyknesse of ye brayne," and powdered rosemary flowers bound to the right arm in a linen cloth "shale make thee light and merrie." Drinking a concoction of rosemary leaves boiled in white wine is said to cure a cough.

And last but not least, according to Gerard, a garland of rosemary worn around the head "comforteth the brain, the memorie, the inward senses, and comforteth the heart and maketh it merry." Whew! This is one herb that is definitely worth a try!

THYME Thymus vulgaris

Thyme is another herb that is drought-tolerant and easy to grow. Another perennial that will also grow as an annual in colder climate zones, thyme likes dryish, well-drained soil and full sun to partial shade. It's a good window box herb. There are a number of different scented thymes, from the standard *T. vulgaris* to the lemon-scented *T. citriodorus* and the caraway-scented *T. herba-barona* variety. Fresh thyme teas and baths are excellent for use in fortifying the systems of both children and adults, and the leafy stalks can be kept in the freezer for winter use. The dried leaves can be used in seasoning meats and vegetables year-round and make an excellent flavoring for stuffing in your Thanksgiving turkey.

The healing, antiseptic qualities of thyme have been appreciated since antiquity and have been used in folk remedies around the world. The Irish drink whey flavored with thyme. The Swiss use the herb in wine and to preserve dried fruit and boil thyme with milk to cure a cough. A Guatemalan folk remedy for coughs and sore throats combines thyme and a chopped onion, boiling them together in water. The mixture is then strained and honey is added before it's drunk.

For herbed meatballs (my kids love these), work a teaspoon each of fresh chopped thyme, chives, marjoram, and parsley into a pound of chopped meat. (For moister meatballs, add an egg and half a cup of breadcrumbs.) Form the meat into balls and roll in flour to which you've added salt and pepper, then fry until well browned.

Other aromatic plants for a garden include lavender, melissa (aka "lemon balm" or "balm mint"), dill, geranium, bay laurel (laurus nobilis), oregano, parsley, lemon verbena, angelica, and yarrow.

Chapter Four

THE TOUCH OF LIFE: AROMATHERAPY AND MASSAGE

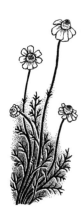

Massage feels good to the hands (and heart) of the person doing the strokes. When we touch, we are touched; we begin to make little miracles happen. We learn to love.

TERESA RAMSEY, *Baby's First Massage*

Aromatherapy and massage are natural companions. In my opinion, aromatic massage is the most pleasurable and effective way of using essential oils. A good massage oil helps speed absorption of the essences through the skin, while heat and friction generated by stroking improve and increase the circulation of blood and lymphatic fluids, helping essential oils to get into the bloodstream faster. The aromatic experience you give is the experience you receive, as the person giving the massage benefits through inhalation of the essences during the massage as well as absorbing massage oil through the hands. All systems can be benefited by stroking the skin, the body's largest organ. Tensions that result from bottled-up emotion and stress can be harmlessly released.

Touch is the first of our senses to develop and, of all our senses, the only one we literally cannot live without. This is powerfully illustrated by the following story from Ashley Montagu's enlightening book *Touching: The Human Significance of the Skin*.

Marasmus, from the Greek meaning "wasting away," was a disease that killed more than half the babies born during the nineteenth century. Even into the 1920s the mortality rate was nearly 100 percent for babies under one or two years of age who were placed in children's institutions in cities throughout the United States. No one expected "foundling" babies to survive. In New York City, their condition was routinely recorded as "hopeless" upon admission, whatever their actual state of health.

Why did this happen? American city hospitals and institutions were well staffed, well equipped, and modern, even state of the art for their time. There was no shortage of food. The children were provided with clothing and a clean bed to sleep in. So why were all the babies dying?

Dr. Montagu links the high incidence of marasmus and the high infant mortality rate of the late nineteenth and early twentieth centuries to child-rearing practices espoused by a Columbia University professor of pediatrics, Dr. Luther Emmet Holt. If you have ever wondered where such concepts as "feeding by the clock" and "letting the baby cry" originally came from, this is the guy.

Holt wrote a booklet called *The Care and Feeding of Children: A Catechism for the Use of Mothers and Children's Nurses*, first published in 1894. It became so influential that it made Holt the Dr. Spock of his time, and his booklet was in its fifteenth printing in 1935. Describing the practice of rocking babies in a cradle as "vicious," Holt's method also condemned demonstrations of affection, such as holding, kissing, and cuddling, as well as quick responses to a child's demands for food or attention. Such overly sentimental behaviors were thought to "spoil" children by making them too dependent on caretakers, whether nurses, nannies, or parents. And so, all across America, health workers and mothers suppressed their "animal" instincts, threw out their cradles and rocking chairs, fed infants according to schedule, regardless of whether or not they were hungry, and "let the baby cry."

Dr. Holt was described by colleagues as a "human machine, austere and unapproachable" and was never known to have said "good morning" to his secretary in all the years she worked for him, nor to have praised anybody or anything. Studies conducted over the last few decades indicate that the child-rearing practices recommended by Holt (if they don't kill the child in the first two years!) will tend to produce human beings quite similar to him—cold, tense, physically restricted, and socially maladjusted.

John Broadus Watson, a professor of psychology at Johns Hopkins University and an earnest devotee of Holt's teachings, published his popular book *Psychological Care of Infant and Child* in 1928. "Never hug and kiss them, never let them sit in your lap," Watson recommended. "If you must, kiss them once on the forehead when they say good night. Shake hands with them in the morning. Give them a pat on the head if they have made an extraordinarily good job of a difficult task. Try it out. In a week's time you will find how easy it is to be perfectly objective with your child." This is a book that was recommended by *Parents Magazine* and *Atlantic Monthly* as a must-have for "every intelligent mother."

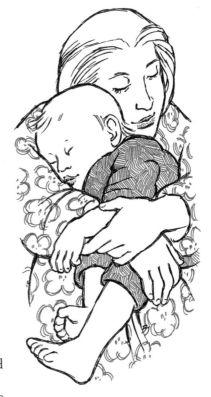

After World War II it became apparent that marasmus was most likely to occur in the "best" homes and institutions, among the most "intelligent" of caretakers. Poorer, less-educated women who had never heard of Watson or Luther Emmet Holt or their philosophy had continued to hold and cuddle their babies, and their children thrived. As the medical establishment got wind of this, changes were gradually made. "Mothering" policies were established in hospitals and institutions, requiring that each baby be picked up and cuddled several times a day. Mortality rates at Bellevue Hospital in New York dropped to under 10 percent by 1938, once "mothering" was instituted in its pediatric wards.

You might think, like I do, that picking up a baby when it cries or feeding a child when the child is hungry is basic common sense. But Holt's teachings are still with us to a certain degree. What mother has not heard a well-meaning relative suggest that she is "spoiling" her baby by holding it too much, or by responding too quickly to an infant's distress? The bottom line is that babies need to be loved, stroked, and held in order to grow up into healthy human beings. A child whose basic needs for touch and love are not met through human contact and interaction with primary caregivers will learn to turn elsewhere for comfort.

Study after study now affirms that babies who are rocked, carried, and kept close to their mother's bodies are biologically and psychologically stronger than infants who don't get continual body contact. Infants who are handled more, cry less, and develop significant advantages in overall health, alertness, and responsiveness on all levels.

Massage and gentle stroking give further advantages, as babies who are stroked by their mothers experience fewer colds and respiratory problems and less vomiting and diarrhea than babies who are not stroked. Positive touch experiences also influence development of the nervous system and immune response. Massage relieves muscle tension, stimulates circulation, improves digestion, and can stimulate production of pain-killing, euphoria-producing chemicals within the body.

Touch is literally what calls us to life. The contractions of labor as a baby exits the uterus and comes down the vaginal canal during birth activate all systems of the body for the increased demands of life outside the womb. The pressure against the skin during delivery helps the infant to get a sense of the boundaries of the physical body, which will later affect self-perception, emotional adjustment, physical coordination, and balance. For these reasons massage is especially important for babies born prematurely or by Caesarean section.

In a fascinating study conducted in 1986 at the Miami Medical Center, twenty premature infants were massaged in fifteen-minute sessions three times a day. A control group of premies received no massage. The babies who were massaged gained 47 percent more weight and were discharged an average of six days earlier than the control group. They were also more active and alert and showed better motor control and neurological development than the nonmassaged babies. Other studies of premature babies receiving stroking and massage have yielded similar results.

Touch is also integral to early bonding experiences. While the primary bonding between mother and infant is established in the first ten minutes following birth, and while the infant "imprints" the bond based on the mother's odor, "there must be supplemental tactile stimulation or this special memory will not become permanently enmeshed in the brain's processes," according to Dr. Michael Leon of the University of California, Irvine. It's the combination of touch and smell that cements the connection between mother and child. This combination can have tremendous influence throughout life.

Children who do not receive appropriate tactile stimulation are much more likely to become violent adults. This seems to be true for human beings regardless of geographic location or culture. James Prescott, a neuropsychologist who studied forty-nine primitive societies, found that in 73 percent of them, the lavishing of physical affection during infancy correlated with low levels of adult violence, while absence of affection for babies corresponded to high levels of violence in adults. The same tendencies are found among Western urban youth.

Touch deprivation and loneliness may also increase the likelihood of later drug abuse. Child psychologists have noted that children who suffer from acute early kinesthetic deprivation experienced increased muscle tension as infants, which can lead to hyperactivity or depression in later childhood.

Touch deprivation and inadequate physical contact have also been linked to skin afflictions, such as infantile eczema, which can persist into adulthood. If we adopt the holistic model and interpret the symptom as an attempt by the body to communicate, this makes perfect sense. The skin is drawing attention to itself and its needs. Many alternative practitioners also link the suppression of childhood eczema through use of cortisone prescriptions with the subsequent development of asthmatic conditions. The repressed symptom simply remanifests in another area of the body if the basic imbalance and unmet need are not addressed.

Other studies indicate that gentle touch can normalize heart rate and rhythm, improve pituitary function (which regulates growth), and generally encourages the development of children who are happier, more self-confident, more cooperative, and loving. Just as a mother who is massaged during pregancy will be more comfortable and adept at stroking her newborn infant, a child whose needs are lovingly met will grow into an adult who is capable of lovingly fulfilling the needs of others.

Essential Oils and Massage

During massage, underlying physiological functions are activated through stimulation of the skin. Stress-relieving and immune-enhancing qualities of both essential oils and massage create a synergy, in which the combination of the two exceeds the effects of either used individually. This is not a new idea. It was Hippocrates who declared in his writings, "The way to health is to have an aromatic bath and scented massage every day."

Following are some suggestions for massage strokes and essential oil combinations that can be used in conjunction with them to relieve certain ailments and discomforts. Don't be intimidated by any difficulty you might have in translating the description into practice—the touch and the feeling that goes with it are much more important than any technique.

Be observant of the cues the recipient of your massage is giving you, and don't be afraid to follow your intuition. Babies and young children will let you know in no uncertain terms if they don't like the way you're touching them! While babies who have been massaged since birth tend to be very relaxed and receptive to receiving a massage, older children for whom it's a new experience might be squirmy or uncomfortable at first. Start with a few minutes at a time to get them used to it. Most kids will sit still for a quick foot or back massage. Once they realize how good it can feel, they'll be requesting more. Even better, they will start to return the favor! How many things in life are sweeter than a shoulder or foot rub offered by tiny hands?

Baby Massage

When a baby is born, a mother is also born.

ASHLEY MONTAGU, *Touching: The Human Significance of the Skin*

Gentle, stroking touch communicates love. It's never too soon to begin massaging your baby. In the Middle Ages it was believed that a newborn infant had to be massaged into proper human form immediately after birth. Babies were then tightly swaddled with rose petals to help "hold" their desired shape. Here in the twentieth century we know that a baby will not turn into an amorphous blob if it isn't stroked right after birth. Yet in a figurative sense there is wisdom and more than a grain of truth in the medieval custom, as so many aspects of being are shaped by early tactile experiences.

Rose essence, in dilution, is the only essential oil I would recommend for use with a newborn baby. Rose is an extremely gentle, "heart-opening" oil whose subtle qualities make it perfectly suited to the happy task of welcoming a new life into the world. Newborn massage with rose opens up baby's new sensory systems in the loveliest possible way, linking the beauty of an exquisite fragrance with the loving touch of parents. Rose also has an affinity for the female reproductive system that can be useful in rebalancing the mother after birth and allaying postpartum depression.

Generally speaking, it's a good idea to avoid the use of fragrance during the period just following birth so as not to interfere with the infant's bonding with the mother via her natural odor and pheromones. Once bonding has occurred, gentle massage with a light nut oil such as sweet almond or sesame with rose (one drop of rose essence to two to four ounces of carrier) can soothe both mother and baby and helps to moisturize dry and peeling newborn skin. In addition, light stroking can improve baby's digestion, which can increase weight gain and enhance overall development. Massage also affects respiration and has a calming effect on the nervous system, which can improve the quality of sleep and ease the transition into life outside the womb.

Newborns sleep a lot and don't have to be awake to be massaged. Stroking a baby before feeding can enhance appetite and digestion. Breastfed babies can be massaged anytime. Babies who are fed formula should not be massaged in the half hour follow-ing a feeding.

Newborn babies chill quite easily. To keep them comfortably warm, the parts of their body not being massaged can be kept covered with a light blanket. A baby can also be stroked through clothing, although then you would obviously not be using a massage oil! If the baby starts to cry during a massage, stop and try to figure out why before you continue. Hunger, a soiled diaper, feeling cold, a too-bright room, overstim-ulation, and tiredness can all cause fussing. Calm the baby on your left shoulder, stroking gently from the head down the back. Walking, rocking, or laying quietly on the warmth of your chest for a few minutes will usually soothe an infant to the point that you can go on with the massage. Or maybe the baby has had enough for now. You can always try again later.

To begin, wash your hands and make sure your nails are well trimmed. Have your massage oil, if you are using it, within easy reach. Set the baby down gently on a padded surface, such as a sheepskin or thick soft blanket. Keep a hand on the baby at all times during the massage to promote a feeling of comfort and security. Before you start stroking, it's a good idea to take a moment to ask if the baby would like a mas-sage. I am not expecting that the baby will answer you! It's simply a gesture of respect for the individuality of the new little being you've brought into the world, and a way of beginning to form an intuitive connection. If you get an intuitive impression that your baby doesn't want to be touched just now, by all means wait for another time.

Warm a bit of oil in your hands—a few drops will do. A newborn's arms and legs are so small that one quick and simple stroke can cover them all.

Form a circle of your right thumb and forefinger (reverse if you're left-handed) around the top of the limb you're stroking and, using a back and forth rocking motion, move down slowly and gently from hip to foot or shoulder to hand. Don't squeeze hard or press—this is a light and gentle "milking" motion. Support the baby's foot (or hand) with your free hand as you do the stroke.

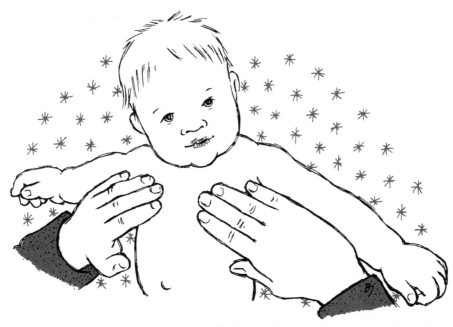

Make sure as you massage that you don't get oil on the baby's hands or fingers. If you do, wipe it off immediately to prevent the baby from rubbing the oil into the eyes. Don't use oil on the baby's face for the same reason.

The back and chest can be stroked slowly and gently from top to bottom with the fingertips. A good stroke for the chest is to put the hands lightly on the center over the sternum and press them lightly in an outward motion toward the sides, as if smoothing the pages of a book. This opens up the breathing and helps clear up any congestion. Also, try making gentle little circles with one or two fingers alongside the spine, moving down. **Never press directly on the spine** of anyone you're giving a massage to, whether a baby, an older child, or an adult, as doing so can throw the spine out of its natural alignment by compressing the vertebrae.

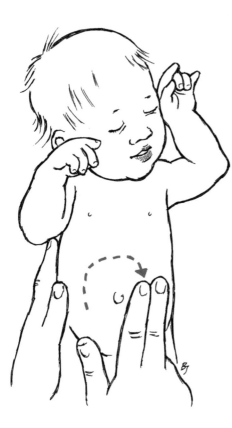

Tracing little circles over the head is soothing to baby too. Use your other hand to support the head as you work. Stroking around the mouth with one finger helps digestion, stimulating the same nerves as does thumb-sucking or a pacifier. To relieve gas or colic, try stroking with two fingers over the digestive area above the umbilical cord, being careful not to get massage oil on the cord itself. Stroke on either side of the umbilical in an "I" shape, then above the cord at a right angle and in an arch, or upside-down "U" shape.

For babies one month or older, try using a drop of stomach-soothing essences of mandarin, tangerine, or clary sage in an ounce of massage oil. Giving the baby a teaspoon of weak chamomile tea or floral water of chamomile or dill can also help.

A good massage pattern to follow for newborn massage is: legs, abdomen, chest, arms, head, and back, finishing up with a return to the legs. The whole process takes only a few minutes and can be repeated several times a day if you wish. Simple stroking prepares you and your child for deeper and more extensive massage techniques that can be learned from classes, or from books such as those listed in the "bibliography" section at the end of this book.

Massaging Older Children

When I was a medical student and my first child was nearly five, he complained so severely about a belly ache that I was worried he might have appendicitis. I asked him to lie down on his bed and sat beside him to examine his belly. As I laid my hand on him to begin to press, he screamed with pain. I asked him if his belly was really that tender, and he said, with tears in his eyes, "No, no, you're sitting on my foot!"

MARY HOWELL, *Healing at Home*

The great thing about massaging older children is that they can tell you where it hurts and what's wrong. Once again, let me stress that techniques are less important than the touch itself. Just pay attention to your child's response. Starting with a relaxation exercise can also improve the effectiveness of your efforts. Here's one that I've used with my kids. They get a big kick out of it, and it teaches them to feel the difference in their own bodies between muscles that are tense and muscles that are relaxed. Have the child lie down, face up on the bed or floor where the massage will take place. I usually start with arms or legs, saying, "Let's see how tense you can make it." The child tenses up, closing the hand into a tight fist, stiffening the elbow, or locking the knee and bringing the foot up rigid. I then "check" for an appropriate level of tension by picking up the limb, shaking it a little to see if it holds the tension, attempting (gently) to bend the joint. Then I say, "Okay, let's see how loose and relaxed you can make it." The object here is to get the limb as loose and floppy as possible. You can repeat the tense/relax testing with each arm and leg, the stomach (tapping gently to check for tension, rubbing or tickling lightly to check relaxation), shoulders, and face. If you're working with more than one child, they tend to turn this into a contest and find the part where you flop their limbs around particularly hilarious.

Sometimes older children will happily be still for a full body massage. Sometimes, especially if you have more than one child, this just isn't possible. Many children (boys especially) go in and out of developmental stages that affect where, how, and how often they are willing to be touched. Taking such things into consideration before you begin can prevent frustration by keeping expectations reasonable. Be patient, be flexible, and remember that even a mere few minutes of a well-timed massage can be beneficial.

Massage can be very comforting and soothing to a child who isn't feeling well, especially when combined with the appropriate essential oils to speed recovery. At bedtime, a few minutes spent stroking the back, chest, and/or soles of the feet with sleep-promoting essences such as lavender or marjoram can help children to let go and make the transition from daytime dynamo to sleeping angel. For working mothers who can't be with their children for most of the day, this can be a special time to be together in a loving way.

Here are a few simple massage strokes that ease anxiety and tension and help speed penetration of essential oils through the skin. These strokes can be used for both children and adults. As with any massage, you'll want to start with clean hands, well-trimmed nails, and a warm, quiet, softly lit room with a padded surface for the child to lie on. Cover with a sheet or light blanket for warmth, and have your oil within easy reach. Keep one hand on the body throughout the massage to maintain a feeling of continuity.

Do not use essential oils in the genital area or near the eyes, as they can cause irritation to sensitive mucous membranes. After an aromatherapy massage you may want to put a T-shirt and socks on the child to keep the oils in contact with the skin so they don't rub off on sheets and bedding.

BACK STROKES

Using flat hands, start at the lower back and move slowly up either side of the spine, pressing gently. When you get to the shoulders, circle out and come back down the sides of the body—one long, continuous stroke. After a minute or so of this, knead the shoulders, squeezing very gently between thumb and fingers with alternate hands. Finish up with raking, spreading the fingers apart and raking the back from top to bottom. You can also make little circles with the fingertips up and down the sides of the spine. And I reiterate, **never press directly on the vertebrae** of anyone you are massaging.

CHEST STROKES

From a position behind the child's head, start with both hands flat, moving down the center of the chest with fingertips pointing toward the feet, then coming back up along the sides of the body, following the same continuous circle you started with on the back. Stroke gently with alternate hands over the heart area.

Coming round to face the child, make clockwise circles over the abdomen with several fingers or the entire hand (depending on the size of the child). Essential oils can be used with this stroke to soothe tummy aches and digestive problems: try tangerine, mandarin, or orange with a drop of clary sage or peppermint (don't use peppermint at bedtime, however—it's too stimulating and may keep your child awake).

To ease coughs and respiratory problems, try this technique from Chinese massage: Have the child sit up, facing you, on your knees or on the edge of a bed or chair. Using a blend containing respiratory-aid essences such as eucalyptus, niaouli, pine, lemon, thyme, chamomile, or peppermint, start at the midline of the chest and stroke outward with the thumbs toward the nipples. Continue for several minutes. Then turn the child around and stroke with the thumbs down along the shoulder blades, from the top of the back to the base of the scapulae for a few minutes more.

According to ancient Eastern medical philosophy, invisible channels of energy called "meridians" run like a highway system all over the body. Illness and emotional stress can cause energy blocks (like traffic jams) to occur along these energy lines. Alternative healing modalities such as acupuncture, acupressure, and shiatsu focus on manipulating certain points along these meridians for the purpose of releasing jammed energy, thereby improving the "flow" and helping to maintain physical harmony. Because all meridians, or energy channels, are said to terminate in the hands and feet, massaging these areas can have a positive influence on internal organs and all systems of the physical body.

Again, *how* you do it is less important than *that* you do it. I can't think of anyone who wouldn't respond favorably to having their feet rubbed. It's deliciously relaxing. Here are a few suggestions for foot massage strokes to add to your repertoire, and some blends to accompany them.

Foot Massage Blends

Included in your kit is a bottle of Lavender Lullaby: A Sleepytime Rainbow Rub. This aromatherapy massage oil blend is specially formulated for use with children and contains the correct dilution of calming, sleep-promoting essential oils (including lavender, geranium, and clary sage) in a carrier base of sweet almond, sesame, and Vitamin E oils. It's a wonderful oil to use with any of the strokes described for children in the massage section. My own children particularly love having it rubbed in with a bedtime foot massage.

Here are some other essential oil combinations you can try: to a half-ounce of carrier oil such as sweet almond or sesame, add a drop of peppermint or rosemary for a stimulating rub. For a calming foot rub try three drops of lavender, chamomile, mandarin or tangerine; or two drops of clary sage, ylang-ylang or rosewood; or one drop rose, jasmine, or neroli. For fever add two drops of lavender, or one drop each of lavender, eucalyptus, and tea tree. For colds add two drops of eucalyptus, myrtle, or niaouli, or one drop of eucalyptus, one drop of benzoin, and one drop of pine. For flu add two drops of ravensara aromatica.

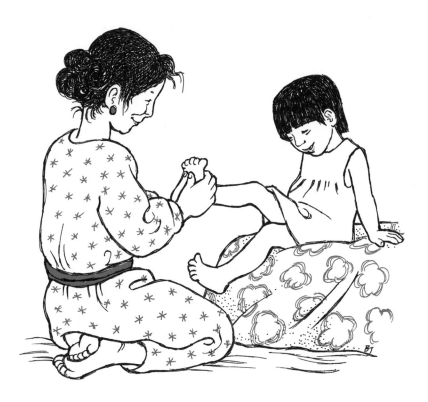

FOOT STROKES

Begin by standing or kneeling near the feet. Placing your hands on them, hold gently for a few moments and take a few deep breaths. Next, put a little oil into your hands and rub them together, warming your palms and oil with the friction. Then put your right hand on the base of the foot, your left hand over the top, and rub the foot briskly for about half a minute. Then, pressing gently on the top of the foot, stretch it toward you, creating a straighter line from the leg down through the toes. Supporting the ankle with one hand, gently rotate the ankle with your other hand, holding near the ball of the foot. Then press gently upward from the ball of the foot toward the knee, exaggerating the right angle of the foot to the leg.

With your fingers loosely curled, rub your knuckles along the bottom of the foot (not too much pressure here—this can tickle!). Next, pull gently on the toes, then rotate each individually.

Pressing with your thumbs, with your fingers over the top of the foot, rub your thumbs up the centerline of the foot from the heel to the ball. When you get to the ball of the foot, your thumbs will separate outward, following the outlines of the bones of the feet. Repeat this several times.

Finish up with a "foot sandwich." Press the foot gently between your palms, your fingers facing toward the ankle and leg, and glide your hands over the entire foot, allowing the "sandwich filling" to slip through.

If your child is sick or has a fever, you may want to try massaging the pressure point

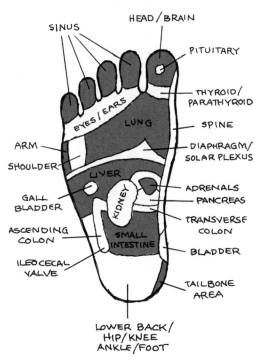

REFLEXOLOGY CHART

BOTTOM OF RIGHT FOOT

SINUS
HEAD / BRAIN
PITUITARY
THYROID/PARATHYROID
EYES / EARS
LUNG
SPINE
ARM
DIAPHRAGM/SOLAR PLEXUS
SHOULDER
LIVER
ADRENALS
GALL BLADDER
KIDNEY
PANCREAS
TRANSVERSE COLON
ASCENDING COLON
SMALL INTESTINE
BLADDER
ILEO CECAL VALVE
TAILBONE AREA
LOWER BACK/ HIP/KNEE ANKLE/FOOT

REFLEXOLOGY CHART

BOTTOM OF LEFT FOOT

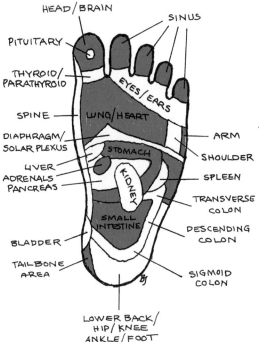

HEAD/BRAIN

SINUS

PITUITARY

THYROID/
PARATHYROID

EYES/EARS

SPINE

LUNG/HEART

DIAPHRAGM/
SOLAR PLEXUS

ARM

STOMACH

SHOULDER

LIVER
ADRENALS
PANCREAS

KIDNEY

SPLEEN

TRANSVERSE
COLON

SMALL
INTESTINE

DESCENDING
COLON

BLADDER

TAILBONE
AREA

SIGMOID
COLON

LOWER BACK/
HIP/KNEE
ANKLE/FOOT

known to the Chinese as *yongquan*, or "bubbling spring." The point is on the sole of the foot, on the centerline near the base of the ball, about a third of the way down between the toes and the heel. Hold the foot with one hand while you massage the point with the thumb of the other hand for a minute or two. Rub in a bit of lavender, eucalyptus, or chamomile to help ease fevers, vomiting, or diarrhea, or generally to cool down a "hot-headed" little one.

Massage for Women

Motherhood brings as much joy as ever, but it still brings boredom, exhaustion and sorrow too. Nothing else ever will make you as happy or as sad, as proud or as tired, for nothing is quite as hard as helping a person develop his own individuality — especially while you struggle to keep your own.

MARGUERITE KELLY AND ELIA PARSONS,
A Mother's Journal

As you begin to incorporate the benefits of aromatic massage into daily life, don't forget yourself! Mothering is a joyful experience, but it's also stressful and demanding. Our acculturation as women, in which a high value is placed on traditionally "feminine" traits such as self-sacrifice and selflessness, combined with the day-to-day realities of motherhood, in which a woman is habitually required to put the needs of others ahead of her own, can create a situation in which we ignore our own needs to the point of burnout and exhaustion. All the "good parenting" knowledge in the world won't help if you're too stressed, too tired, or too frazzled to apply it! Even mothers need mothering from time to time.

Ask a spouse, partner, family member, or friend to trade massage sessions with you, or build in time for yourself to visit a bodyworker regularly. Any time or money you spend on bodywork is a long-term investment in your good health and peace of mind.

STRESS RELIEF

Included in your kit is a bottle of Stress Relief massage oil, a blend containing essential oils specifically chosen to help ease stress and rebalance the female system. Essences of lavender, eucalyptus, and geranium are blended in a skin-nourishing carrier base of hazelnut, sweet almond, sesame, and Vitamin E oils. Use it with the following strokes, or anytime you need a release from accumulated tension. Because continuous stress can erode the body's natural defenses, I use Stress Relief daily as a preventive to keep my vitality high and my resistance intact.

Nervous tension invariably manifests in tense, tight muscles in the head, neck, and shoulders. Often tension headaches can be alleviated merely by releasing and relaxing this area. The nice thing about this set of techniques is that they can be performed anywhere. While it's wonderful to be able to take your clothes off and lie down to receive a massage, it's not always practical.

These strokes concentrate on the neck, shoulders, spine, and base of the skull. The heat of the hands and friction from the massage help speed penetration of the essential oils into the many blood vessels and nerves radiating out from the spinal area.

Neck and Shoulder Strokes

Begin by taking a moment to ground your energy with the energy of the person you're massaging. While the person sits facing away from you, lay your hands on her shoulders, leaning in slightly to create a mild downward pressure for a few moments. This is soothing and allows the recipient of the massage to get accustomed to the feeling of your touch. Take a few deep breaths, and encourage your partner to do likewise.

Begin with a simple kneading of the trapezius, the muscle that runs along the top of the shoulder. With your thumb on the back and your fingers in front, gently squeeze and lift the muscle. The movement is toward the spine, then lifting slightly. Gradually you'll feel the muscle begin to loosen under your hand.

Then move on to loosen the back of the neck. Support the forehead with your free hand so the weight of the head is resting in your palm, to encourage the neck muscles to release. Then cup the hand and place it across the back of the neck starting where the neck meets the shoulders and moving upward to the base of the skull, squeezing on either side of the spinal column. Pressure on the side of the neck being pressed by the heel of the hand will be different from the side being squeezed by the fingers, so be sure to switch hands to keep it symmetrical.

Once the back of the neck is softened, you can use the thumb to facilitate further release. Support the forehead now with your free forearm and, moving in a line parallel to the spine, start at the base of the neck and move upward. You'll feel a kind of groove or space between the bones of the spine and where the (usually tense and knotted!) muscle mass begins. This is the channel where you want to begin. As you go along, you'll also feel slight indentations in the channel, and those are the places where you want to apply pressure with the thumb. Start with very mild pressure, as tension held in this area can make it very sore and sensitive. Ask for feedback as you go along to make sure that what you're doing feels good to the recipient and isn't causing undue discomfort or pain. When you've reached the base of the skull, change sides.

Move out about an inch from where you started with the thumb pressure points and do another row up, again feeling for the indentations. Along with mild pressure you can also move the thumb in little circles. Change and do the other side.

Again supporting the forehead with your forearm, use your thumb to press into points along the base of the skull bone, or occiput. Start in the hollow just to the side of where the spinal column meets the skull, and work out along the bottom of the bone. The action of the pressure is in and slightly upward.

You can finish up with another round of kneading to the trapezius area, which by now should be much looser than when you started.

Back Strokes

If it's possible to do so, you can use thumb pressure strokes and circles all down the back in the channel that runs alongside the spine and in a second channel between the spine and the scapula (shoulder blade). If the recipient is seated for this, you'll want to support the chest with your forearm as you apply thumb pressure along the points. And, of course, do both sides.

Following are some strokes that are excellent for releasing lower back tension and the congested feeling that often accompanies menstruation. These strokes can also be used to alleviate the pain of menstrual cramps and to release tension and encourage contractions during labor. **Do not use these strokes during pregnancy**.

The sacrum is full of nerve endings and blood vessels that affect the pelvic area and is another wonderful absorption point for essential oils. Try using back strokes and sacral release strokes with massage blends containing essential oils such as lavender, clary sage, fennel, grapefruit, geranium, and lemongrass. Laboring mothers will enjoy a blend containing confidence-building jasmine, which also encourages contractions, as does clary sage.

Sitting at the recipient's head and facing her feet, begin with a firm but gentle elliptical back stroke, moving down along either side of the spine with the fingers pointing toward the buttocks, then coming gently back up along the sides of the body. After several strokes, move your hands to the base of the spine and rest them there for a moment before locating the first points on the sacrum.

Sacrum Release Strokes

The sacrum is an area that extends in an inverted triangle from a point originating at the coccyx, or tailbone, extending upward toward the lower back. Start by finding two hollow points on either side of the backbone, along the top flat side of the triangle. Use your thumbs to press into these points using a gentle but firm pressure, and hold the position for thirty to sixty seconds.

Now come around to sit on one side or the other of the back, facing toward the head of the recipient. You'll be working on the side you're sitting on, doing strokes on this half of the back, then changing position to repeat the process on the other side. In your mind, think of the sacrum as two triangles joined by the spine. Using light pressure, stroke gently with the thumbs in tiny, alternating strokes from the spine moving outward toward the sides of the body. It's a kind of chaining or braiding action.

Next, find the channel right alongside the spine and feel for the indentations, or pressure points, applying firm pressure and little circles with the thumb. Follow the pressure points up to the midback area.

Use your thumbs to depress a second row of points, this time on the rise of the muscle parallel to the backbone. Continue the points up to the midback.

Now rest your hand gently on the buttocks, on the cheek that is on the same side as you are sitting. Squeezing slightly and pressing in with the heel of your hand, knead around the buttocks in a full circle to release any tension being held there. The action is similar to what a cat does when it's preparing to lie down someplace soft and comfortable.

Moving up toward the sacrum, use thumb pressure on points along the base of sacrum, starting at the coccyx and moving outward along the edge of the bone, pressing in and slightly up, the same movement you used at the base of the skull in the stress-reliever massage.

Knead the buttocks in another full circle.

Then, with the palms flat against the back and alongside the spine, press firmly (keeping the entire hand in contact with the skin) and slide up toward the top of the back in a single strong stroke. Repeat on the same side with the other hand, alternating hands with firm and continuous stroking pressure. This is a very comforting and grounding stroke and helps to redistribute the trapped tension and energy liberated through manipulation of the sacral area.

Move to the other side of the body and repeat all the same strokes. Then return to the position at the top of the recipient's head, and repeat the back stroke a few more times.

Women in labor can be massaged with the same strokes as they sit up or lie on their sides. Pressure against the sacrum can provide a welcome sense of relaxation and relief during labor and contractions. The aroma of the essences is soothing and comforting, especially in unfamiliar surroundings such as a hospital or birthing room.

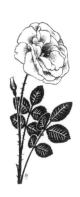

Chapter Five

CHILDREN AND AROMATHERAPY

What has happened to childhood?
PRESIDENT BILL CLINTON

It's a tough time to be a kid. The staggering complexity and frenetic pace of urban-oriented, media-saturated modern life have drastically altered the experience of childhood. The result: stress and an overall deterioration of our children's health, fitness, and ability to cope.

What forms of stress can a child be subject to? First, there are the ordinary stressors of childhood associated with developmental milestones, sibling conflicts, family problems, moving, and starting school. These are further augmented by sociological conditions, such as the changing configuration of the family due to high divorce rates. The amount of time parents spend with their children has been cut almost in half in the last thirty years. The bulk of that lost time is being made up by childcare workers—a profession second only to gas station attendants in turnover rate—and TV and video games—sedentary activities characterized by steady streams of violent images. With 70 percent of our population now living in urban areas, fresh air and sunshine are not always part of a child's daily play experiences. A fourth grader is quoted in *Sierra* magazine as saying, "I like to play indoors better 'cause that's where all the electrical outlets are."

Support and guidance once provided by the nuclear and extended families may be minimal or not available at all, putting an incredible emotional strain on children. Add to this a poor diet, environmental contamination, and a shaky economy and it's no wonder that more than a third of American children suffer from stress-related health problems at some point.

The statistics are truly alarming. One out of five American kids now lives well below the poverty level, with accompanying substandard care and the risk of developing long-term problems such as failure in school, teenage pregnancy, drug abuse, and criminal behavior. Since 1971, prescriptions for the drug Ritalin, used to treat hyperactivity, increased more than sixfold. American children have the highest incidence of heart disease in the world, with asthma vying for second place as the most prevalent chronic condition. One in ten American kids is afflicted with severe allergies. Childhood cancer, once a rarity recorded in medical journals, is now the leading cause of natural death in youngsters under the age of fifteen, its incidence having increased by almost 200 percent since 1900. Birth defects have tripled in the last twenty-five years.

Despite this grim reality and the bewildering array of external forces that seem beyond our ability to influence or control, there are many things we parents can do to keep ourselves and our children as strong and healthy as possible. We can strive to maintain a clean and healthy diet. It's likely that if we're eating well, our children will be too. We can model for them a physically active life and respect for the natural environment. We can choose to live according to ethics and principles of tolerance and community involvement. We can show them, by example, how to jump off the merry-go-round and relax from time to time, to stop and smell the roses, or the rose essence, if you will!

Aromatherapy and the use of essential oils can help in an emotional and spiritual sense to reawaken our children's natural connection to the living world. A recent study indicated that for people born prior to 1970, natural smells predominate in association with childhood memories. But for those born after 1970, their most beloved odors tend to be synthetic in origin, such as the smells of Play-Doh and crayons. How can we expect our children to have a reverence for and interest in preserving a world they've never experienced? It's important for us to remind our kids, and ourselves, that we have a place in the vast and fragile web of life on Earth. If we turn to Nature for help when we need it, perhaps Nature will also be able to turn to us. The development of a healthy relationship between human beings and the planet we live on is essential at this point in our history to ensure our mutual survival.

Essential oils also provide an attractive alternative in the treatment of many common childhood ailments. Unlike antibiotics, the use of which tends to undermine a child's natural health, certain essences can actually bolster immune response. And as the following story from my own experience illustrates, as childhood stress-relievers, essential oils truly can't be beat.

In the aftermath of last year's earthquake in Los Angeles, both my children developed problems with sleeping. Nightly aftershocks weren't helping matters any! My son Nick, then seven, came home one day and asked me to buy him some sleeping pills he'd seen on a TV commercial. "You just take one at night and you wake up in the morning feeling refreshed!" he told me. (Talk about the power of advertising!) He was highly doubtful at first when I told him we could get the same results with a cup of chamomile tea and an aromatherapy massage.

I made a special oil for him—a rose blend sedative that was more potent than our usual lavender bedtime rub. When he was finished with his tea, I massaged the sedative into his feet, back, and chest, watching as his eyes started to droop. Mustering just enough energy to register slight surprise he sighed, "Wow, Mom. I guess it really…works…" He went to sleep before he finished the sentence, slept through that night's aftershock, and woke up in the morning, "feeling refreshed"!

You can use essential oils with children in much the same way you would use them on yourself or another adult: in the bath, in a diffusor, in compresses, in perfume oils, and in massage. Because children are smaller and their skin is more sensitive and permeable than that of adults, you'll want to be careful about which oils you choose and the dilution at which you use them. For babies under one year of age, a single drop of essential oil is usually an adequate dose (never neat on the skin). For children aged one to five years, three or four drops will be plenty in a bath. Depending on the essences used, massage oils for older children may contain up to fifteen drops of essential oil to an ounce of carrier oil. It's always best to start with a low dilution until you become familiar with how your child interacts with various essences — everyone is unique in this regard. Watch carefully for any signs of discomfort or skin irritation before increasing the dose.

The following essential oils are generally recognized as safe to use on children in the appropriate dilutions:

lavender	Roman chamomile	blue chamomile
geranium	eucalyptus	pine (never neat on skin)
niaouli	tea tree	mandarin/tangerine
orange	lemon	peppermint (a drop or less)
rose	rosewood	rosemary
clary sage	ylang-ylang	neroli
jasmine	dill	thyme linalol

Sweet almond oil and sesame oil are excellent carriers for children's massage blends. You can also use hazelnut, safflower, grapeseed, or canola oils, with a bit of wheat germ oil or Vitamin E added to prevent rancidity. Olive oil and unrefined sesame oil tend to have strong odors that children don't particularly like. Castor oil, which has been shown to increase immunoglobulin production, is a thick, heavy oil that can be added to provide up to a third of your carrier. Evening primrose and *Rosa rubignosa* (aka *Rosa mosqueta* or rose hip seed oil) also make excellent additions due to their high fatty acid content and regulatory action on underlying physiological functions. In Europe, evening primrose and rosa rubignosa are used to treat hyperactivity.

Never use strong essential oils such as savory, thyme (except for linalol chemotype), oregano, sage, or cinnamon on children for compresses, bath, or massage (they could be used in the diffusor). The smaller and more sensitive the child, the milder the oil should be. For extremely sensitive children, stick to the gentlest oils, such as lavender, chamomile, mandarin, rosewood, clary sage, rose, and neroli. Other oils from the above list can be used in the diffusor or vaporizer, or in a bowl of hot water placed next to the bed.

Aromatherapy for Babies

It's funny how babies who sleep so much in the hospital seem to wake up just in time to go home! Those early months of infancy can be extremely challenging as new moms and dads figure out how to balance their own needs with the demands of caring for a newborn. My personal nomination for the most stressful situation in life is to be awake at 3 A.M. holding a wailing newborn infant who will not be comforted no matter what you do. Once you've checked out the obvious possibilities, such as a soiled diaper, hunger, and too much or too little clothing, the next most likely candidates are loneliness and colic. Loneliness is generally comforted by walking, rocking, and cuddling. If wailing persists, it's probably colic.

Make a mental note of what you ate that day (if you're breast-feeding) to check for a possible connection between what has gone into your breast milk and your baby's distress. (My children both ended up with middle-of-the-night colic whenever I ate tomatoes or other highly acidic foods.) Then, by all means, try some of the abdominal massage techniques listed in the massage chapter. You can also add a drop of essential oil to a bowl of steaming water placed near the baby's crib. Chamomile, lavender, dill, tangerine or mandarin, and clary sage are all helpful for digestive upsets. A teaspoon of weak chamomile tea or floral water of chamomile or neroli (orange blossom) can also help.

To promote sleep, a drop of Roman chamomile or lavender can be put into a bowl of steaming water in baby's room. Orange is a wonderful daytime oil to diffuse in the nursery, and babies really seem to enjoy it.

You can make a lovely mobile to hang over your child's crib or bassinette that will provide visual stimulation while scenting the room and having aromatherapeutic effects. Make some small figures or shapes from scraps of cotton, silk, or other "breathable" cloth, and fill them with dried aromatic herbs such as lavender and chamomile flowers to which you've added a few drops of essential oils. For newborns, black-and-white fabric designs catch the eye and stimulate brain function while strengthening the eye muscles. Next, form a circular hoop of wire (an old clothes hanger will do) and tie on cording at the four compass points, knotting it into a loop at the top to allow it to hang from a ceiling hook. Thread a needle with plastic thread or fishing line and run it through the top of the stuffed shapes you've made, tying the other end to the wire hoop. (Space the figures evenly so that the hoop hangs straight.) The movement of air in the room will make the suspended figures dance, and the scent of the dried herbs and essences will waft delightfully over bassinette or crib, stimulating your baby's developing olfactory circuits as well.

Try making up a blend of equal parts lavender, tea tree, and eucalyptus for all-purpose cleaning and disinfecting of children's areas, diaper pails, and so on. Add ten drops of this blend to a sprayer full of water, shake vigorously, and spritz around the room at least once a day. The essential oil mist will do away with airborne pathogens, then settle onto rugs, carpets, and other surfaces to continue their antiseptic, antiviral, and antifungal actions. A few drops of this blend is also a good addition to the final rinse water for babies' clothes and diapers.

Dry, peeling, newborn skin responds well to rose. Or try using blue chamomile or lavender, in a skin-nourishing oil base of hazelnut, with a little bit of wheat germ, carrot seed, or evening primrose. One of the few things you can't use lavender for is cradle cap. Instead, try massaging in a drop of geranium or eucalyptus citriodora diluted in sweet almond or sesame oil after the bath.

For baby's colds or respiratory problems, diffuse eucalyptus or the combination mentioned above of lavender, tea tree, and eucalyptus. A drop of eucalyptus (*smithii* variety) can also be added to the bath for babies over six months old. Swish your hand through the water to disperse the essences before putting the baby in. Generally speaking, essential oils can be irritating to the eyes, so make sure not to splash the bathwater near the baby's face, and avoid getting it on the baby's hands, which could come into contact with the eyes.

Adding a drop of lavender or chamomile to the bath can help prevent diaper rash by inhibiting the growth of bacteria and fungus on the skin.

Aromatherapy and Common Childhood Ailments

COLDS AND RESPIRATORY CONDITIONS

Eucalyptus, used by itself or in conjunction with other oils such as pine, tea tree, niaouli, lavender, thyme, and peppermint, helps to open up the lungs and ease breathing. Try it in the vaporizer or diffusor, in steam inhalations, in baths, in massage oils, or put a drop on a cotton ball tucked into the pillowcase to fight colds and encourage deep breathing during sleep. Eucalyptus oil is mucolytic and expectorant and has been shown to penetrate the lungs when rubbed into the skin. Eucalyptus also kills invading microorganisms as they enter the body. This makes it a superior form of treatment in colds and flu, where the use of antibiotics to rid the body of bacterial infections has no effect whatsoever against the virus that caused the illness in the first place. Eucalyptus is antibacterial as well. A simple 2 percent solution of eucalyptus has been demonstrated to kill more than 70 percent of airborne staphylococci bacteria.

A eucalyptus/lavender/tea tree blend should be diffused in a sickroom in a diffusor or vaporizer to purify and disinfect the air, thereby preventing the spread of infection to other family members. Eucalyptus deepens the breathing, oxygenating the body and providing overall enhancement of vitality and immune support. Massage an oil containing eucalyptus, alone or with lavender, into the soles of the feet to bring down a fever or put a child to sleep. It's also great for soothing tired or overworked muscles and joints and has been used to treat diabetes and hypoglycemia by helping to balance blood sugar. Eucalyptus can be used topically in dilution to help heal herpes of all types, including chicken pox and shingles. The oil also repels lice and fleas.

There are over three hundred varieties of eucalyptus in existence, the most commonly available being *Eucalyptus globulus. E. globulus* is excellent for respiratory and sinus complaints, particularly when the infection is deeply lodged in the lungs. However, don't put the diffusor too close to a child's bed when using this oil, or it may stimulate a coughing reflex if the oil is too closely breathed.

E. australiana is good for throat problems and general lung cleansing. *E. citriodora*, or "eucalyptus lemon," can be used for summer colds, general detoxification, and to repel insects. It has a calming, soothing effect. *E. dives*, or "eucalyptus peppermint," and *E. polybractae* both have high ketone contents that make them unsuitable for use with children. They should also be avoided by pregnant women. Try instead the variety *E. radiata* for respiratory congestion and sinus conditions. *E. radiata* is best for steam inhalations and the diffusor since it will not overstimulate the coughing reflex. The extremely gentle *E. smithii*, which is so mild it is said not to cause eye irritation, is a particularly effective preventive during cold season that can be used undiluted on the body if necessary. It's also the best eucalyptus to use on tired, aching muscles.

Chamomile is another excellent oil to use in rubs and inhalations for respiratory and bronchial complaints, as is rosemary (*cineole* variety). Try a blend of rosemary, lavender, and chamomile to massage over the chest, back, and ribs. A combination of sunny orange and highly antiseptic cinnamon essence makes a wonderful diffusor blend to use as a preventive during cold season, but don't use this blend for bath or massage as it would irritate the skin.

The warming properties of sesame oil make it a particularly good carrier oil for cold and respiratory massage blends. Add castor oil for its immune-enhancing properties. A warm bath before a massage helps to bring the blood to the surface, promoting more rapid absorption of the essential oils. It's nice if you can heat your massage oil gently, especially before a bedtime massage. Thickly apply the blend, using some of the respiratory relief strokes described in the massage chapter, and don't be too concerned about the oil soaking in. You can cover your child with one or two T-shirts after rubbing the back and chest, then massage the feet with the same oil and cover the feet with socks before tucking in. Quick action on your part at the first sign of discomfort can often nip a cold or flu in the bud.

Use your respiratory blend as a preventive throughout cold season by rubbing a little into the back and chest before sending your child to school or preschool. Fresh or fresh frozen thyme tea is a good all-round fortifier. At the first sign of excess mucus, eliminate mucus-increasing foods such as dairy products, orange juice, bananas, and brown rice from the child's diet. Make sure your child gets plenty of sleep and avoid overstimulating activities until the threat of impending illness is well past.

Fever

My children have responded very well to a lukewarm bath with a few drops of lavender, which I've found can have a dramatic effect on bringing down high temperatures. The child will probably cry at first upon being put into the tub, since even lukewarm water will feel cold to a child in a feverish state. Try a foot massage or lukewarm compresses to the feet with lavender and/or eucalyptus. **Don't use cold water on a feverish child!** The cold will constrict the blood vessels, keeping the heat in and making your child even more upset and uncomfortable. For fevers brought on by overexcitement and overstimulation, chamomile can also be a good choice. Put a drop of chamomile or lavender on the thumb when massaging the yongquan pressure point in the foot as described in Chapter Four.

Fever should not be indiscriminately suppressed. It's the body's natural way of combating invading organisms that can't live in the elevated body temperature. However, extremely high temperatures can lead to convulsions, and professional help should be sought under such circumstances.

CALMING AND SLEEP

To promote a soothing, relaxed atmosphere, try diffusing a blend of lavender and mandarin or tangerine in the bedroom for a few minutes before your child goes in to sleep. Essential oils are also a perfect addition to any bedtime ritual when used in the bath or in massage. A warm bath with a couple of drops of lavender, chamomile,

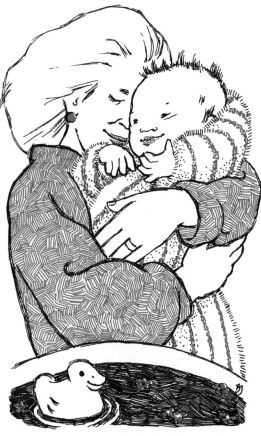

mandarin, or benzoin, or even a single drop of a precious essence such as rose, jasmine, or neroli, can drain a child's tensions away. Follow up with an aromatic massage in bed using any of the same sleep-inducing essences diluted in a carrier.

A drop of essential oil on the pillow can also be comforting. (Be careful with essences such as tangerine or rose absolute, which can stain white or light-colored pillowcases.) My kids love their "sleep pillows," which we make from scraps of muslin and old silk skirts and blouses. Simply cut two small rectangles of muslin, sew them together on three sides, stuff them with a mixture of dried lavender and chamomile blossoms (and a few hops, if your children like the smell), then sew up the top. We make a slipcover from silk scraps, sewing a finished border around the top edges after sewing seams along the other three sides, just like a little pillowcase. You can get as elaborate as you want with this, embroidering the slipcover with the child's name or favorite fairy-tale images. At bedtime, scrunch the sleep pillow between your hands to release the soothing aroma of the volatile oils. The fragrance can be freshened up from time to time by putting drops of essential oil on the muslin inner pillow. The outer silk cover can be hand-washed as necessary. A sleep pillow for the cold season can be made using pine needles for stuffing and essences of eucalyptus, pine, balsam fir (which smells like a Christmas tree), or the lavender/tea tree/eucalyptus combination to intensify the healing benefits. Dried rose petals, alone or mixed with lavender, also make a nice filling.

EARACHE AND SORE THROATS

Never pour any blend of essential oils into the ears. At the first sign of discomfort, put a drop of lavender onto a cotton swab and apply it very gently inside the ear. Warm some carrier oil, such as sesame or sweet almond, and add to it a drop of clary sage or chamomile, then massage gently around the outside of the ear and down along the neck and shoulders. My children take a while to sit still for this treatment, but patience and persistence eventually pay off, and I've found it very effective.

If the earache is related to a secondary infection in the throat or is part of a cold or flu, you'll also want to include highly antiseptic and antibacterial oils like eucalyptus, thyme linalol, tea tree, niaouli, and lemon in gentle massage over the lymph glands of the neck and armpits and into the shoulders, chest, and back. Repeat every two to three hours, unless the child is sleeping, in which case it's better to allow the child to rest.

Cypress is the most effective essential oil I've used for treating a sore throat. If you manage to catch it at the first sign of discomfort, sometimes a single drop can do the trick. The best way to apply it is to put a drop on a cotton swab and apply it directly to the back of the throat (this can be next to impossible to accomplish with some youngsters!). Tea tree is also effective, as is lavender massaged into the neck and throat area for that "ticklish" feeling that sometimes precedes a full-blown sore throat.

Even when antibiotics are prescribed for ear and throat infections, don't hesitate to use aromatherapy to help speed the process of recovery. Using the essences can help bolster the body's natural immune response and prevent the cycle of dependence on antibiotics for ear infection control which I have seen go on for years with some children, to the detriment of their basic health.

SKIN PROBLEMS

Lavender, which stimulates cell growth and regeneration, is generally the first choice for most childhood skin care needs, such as burns, bites, scrapes, and scratches. Blue chamomile is an excellent anti-inflammatory essential oil and takes the itch and discomfort right out of insect bites, such as those from fleas or mosquitoes. For rashes and cuts, lavender and geranium speed healing. Childhood eczema responds well to lavender and chamomile, especially when the essences are diluted in a high grade carrier oil containing up to 10 percent jojoba or hazelnut, with a little Vitamin E and evening primrose or rosa mosqueta.

BUMPS AND BRUISES

Hematomas and sprains can be greatly alleviated with compresses of lavender and helichrysum. Blue chamomile is an excellent choice if the injury is accompanied by heat and swelling. A drop of lavender can be applied neat (undiluted) to bruises to speed healing.

GROWING PAINS

Leg aches are common in children over five due to overexercise and rapid growth. A warm soak in the tub followed by a brisk leg massage works wonders and can also help prevent those middle-of-the-night charley horse cramps. Rosemary has long been used by marathon runners to warm up and cool down. It can be used alone or in combination with lavender and lemongrass to make a friction rub for overworked muscles. Eucalyptus (particularly *E. smithii*), tea tree, juniper, and birch can help as well.

TUMMY UPSETS

Clockwise massage of the abdomen and the strokes listed in the massage chapter, used in tandem with essences such as tangerine, mandarin, clary sage, and peppermint, can help alleviate gas, colic, and tummy aches. Orange essence helps diarrhea, as does diluted lemonade. Also, herbal teas of chamomile, fennel, or peppermint, fresh or dried, soothe stomach upsets, as does chewing on dried fennel seeds.

PARTIES, MOODS, AND BABYSITTERS

Have you ever gotten dressed for an evening out, only to have your child cling to your leg like a koala to a gum tree as you attempted to walk out the door? Are your kids prone to sudden fits of obstinacy that coincide with when you absolutely must be somewhere, five minutes ago? These are the times to use the Happy Bath for Cranky Kids that comes with your kit! Happy Bath contains oils of tangerine and clary sage that are simultaneously euphoric and soothing. A well-timed calming bath or massage, given just before the onset of potentially stressful situations can often head trouble off at the pass. To give yourself a well-deserved break and cause others to marvel at your child's equanimity under duress, try the following.

Tantrum Creme
4 oz. sesame oil
4 oz. sweet almond oil
1 oz. beeswax
8 oz. rose or chamomile or lavender floral water
A few drops evening primrose or rosa mosqueta
2 drops clary sage
2 drops ylang-ylang
2 drops lavender
6 drops tangerine or mandarin

In a bain marie or double boiler, heat the sesame and sweet almond oil together, then add the beeswax and stir until completely melted. Remove from heat. Warm the floral water to room temperature or higher and drizzle into the oil and beeswax mixture, beating constantly until cool.

Add the evening primrose or rosa mosqueta. Add the essential oils last to prevent evaporation. Pour into jars or squeeze-top bottles. Rub into the skin of the arms, legs, feet, back, or chest.

Don't forget to use your diffusor on such occasions as well. Any of the citruses create a cheerful atmosphere, and you can always count on lavender or clary sage to relax and uplift. Ylang-ylang, which soothes hypertension and calms anger, fear, and nervous tension blends well with orange. Tangerine is a good mood enhancer, with a drop of peppermint for a fresh perky scent that kids love. Eucalyptus is a good balancer, especially in combination with lavender and anxiety-reducing lemon. Geranium eases nervous tension and can be combined with rose, lavender, benzoin, or clary sage.

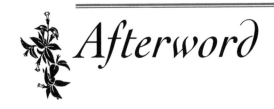

Afterword

Children are our most precious resources. In them reside our hopes and wishes, and our ability to influence the future. All children deserve to grow up happy and healthy, with an abundance of fond and joyful childhood memories to start them on their way in life. I hope you will use the information contained in this book to enhance your experience of mothering, and to create many beautiful moments and memories that you and your child will always share.

It's never too late to have a happy childhood!

Safety Information

The oils suggested for use in the text of this book, are generally recognized as safe to use in accordance with specified instructions in the appropriate dilutions. (See recommended dilutions in Chapter Three.) There are more than 200 essential oils currently available in the marketplace, the bulk of which are used by the flavoring, fragrancing, and pharmaceutical industries. Not all of these essential oils are suitable to use for aromatherapeutic purposes. **Never** use an essential oil without being fully knowledgeable regarding its purity, its purpose, its safety, and its proper application.

While internal usage is sometimes practiced in Europe under medical supervision, it is not advocated by this author due to possible damage to internal organs as a result of improper use. High internal dosages of certain essential oils can cause convulsions, kidney and liver damage, miscarriage, and, with certain toxic oils, death. Keep your oils stored out of the reach of children, and use only pure, aromatherapy-grade essential oils sold by reputable suppliers such as those listed in the Resource Guide at the end of this book.

The following oils are **toxic** and should never be used for aromatherapy:

Boldo	Mustard	Horseradish
Wormseed	Mugwort	Pennyroyal
Calamus	Thuja	Wormwood
Bitter Almond	Savin	Tansy
Rue	Wintergreen	Cornmint
Savory	Ajowan	Buchu
Sassafras	Camphor	

In addition to the oils listed above, the following oils should also be avoided during pregnancy:

Basil	Bay Laurel	Clove
Myrrh	Birch	Origanum
Marjoram	Tarragon	Thyme

The following oils are very irritating to the skin and should not be used in bath or massage:

Clove	Cinnamon	Cassia
Origanum		

The following oils are potentially irritating to mucus membranes, such as the mouth, respiratory tract, and genitourinary tract. Discontinue using these oils in bath or massage if irritation results.

Thyme	Peppermint	Spearmint
Bay Laurel		

The following oils are phototoxic and can cause permanent pigment discoloration:

Bergamot (except for bergapteneless)		Lemon Lime
Bitter Orange	Angelica	Cumin
Opoponax	Verbena	

The following oils should be used sparingly to prevent dermal sensitization in highly sensitive individuals. If irritation occurs, discontinue use.

Citronella	Geranium (Reunion)	
Ginger	Litsea	Cubeba
Pine (dwarf or scotch)	Terebinth	Peru Balsam
Benzoin Resinoid	Bay Laurel	Costus
Ylang-Ylang		

Quick Reference Guide to Essential Oils

Following is a quick reference guide to the essential oils mentioned in this book, including botanical names, country of origin, healing properties, traditional applications and precautions.

Basil: *Ocimum basilicum*
France, Reunion
Properties: Antispasmodic; tonic; stimulating; aphrodisiac (This may be legend, as it was given to horses and asses during mating season to stimulate desire.)
Physical Applications: Headaches; migraines; colds and runny nose (restores sense of smell); chest infections; bronchitis; whooping cough; vertigo; scanty or painful periods; muscle exhaustion; wasp stings and snakebites (first aid, essence or bruised leaves)
Subtle Applications: Mental fatigue; clarity; opening the mind; anxiety; melancholy
Precautions: Use sparingly, can be irritating to the skin

Benzoin: *Styrax benzoin*
Thailand
Properties: Stimulates circulation; aids respiration; soothes irriated skin; reduces nervous tension
Physical Applications: Colds; flu; cough; sore throats; chapped skin; chilblains; stomach pains; urinary tract infections

Subtle Applications: Warming; soothing; anxiety; loneliness; depression

Bergamot: *Citrus aurantium bergamia*
Italy
Properties: Antispasmodic; antiseptic; increases photosensitivity; vermifuge
Physical Applications: Colic; acne; oily/infected skin; cystitis/urethritis; eczema; vaginal pruritis or discharge; insect repellent; chickenpox; shingles; cold sores; intestinal parasites; appetite stimulant; digestive aid
Subtle Applications: Depression; tension; anxiety
Precautions: Do not use before going out in the sun. Can cause permanent pigment discoloration.

Birch: *Betula lenta*
United States
Properties: Diuretic; lymphatic and blood purifier; analgesic
Physical Applications: Cellulitis; water retention; arthritis; rheumatism; kidney and urinary tract ailments

Carrot Seed: *Daucus carota*
France
Properties: Cleansing; purifying; draining; tonic; stimulates elasticity
Physical Applications: Dark spots and blemishes; aged skin; wrinkles; itching; dryness; dermatitis; skin rashes; psoriasis; eczema

Cedarwood: *Cedrus atlantica* (atlas cedar)
Morocco
Properties: Antiseptic; mucolytic; astringent; tonic; digestive stimulant; sedative; aphrodisiac
Physical Applications: Cystitis; vaginal discharge; chronic bronchitis; respiratory conditions; acne; dandruff; scalp problems; repels insects

Subtle Applications: Stress; tension; deep relaxation; meditation
Precautions: Do not use during pregnancy.

Chamomile: *Anthemis nobilis (*Roman*)*
France, Hungary
Properties: Antispasmodic; anti-inflammatory; analgesic; urinary tract disinfectant
Physical Applications: Colic and digestive cramps in children; teething (in infants); headache; loss of appetite; infantile diarrhea; fever (due to overexcitement and nerves); ulcers; lower backache (lumbar region); conjunctivitis; inflamed eyelids; fevers (due to nervous conditions); irregular or painful periods; excess menstrual bleeding; PMS, nausea; sensitive or dry skin; dermatitis; eczema; allergies; earache
Subtle Applications: Calming; soothing; shock; grief; insomnia; hysteria; neurasthenia; hypersensitivity; irritability; antidepressant

Chamomile, German or Blue: *Matricaria chamomilla*
Morocco
Properties: Anti-inflammatory; analgesic; immunostimulant; healing
Physical Applications: Muscle aches; sensitive or inflamed skin; allergies; itching; herpes; boils; sores; rheumatic pains; arthritis; headache; insomnia; colic; teething pain; digestive problems; female reproductive system
Subtle Applications: Anger; tantrums; irritability

Clary sage: *Salvia sclarea*
France, Spain, Australia
Properties: Antispasmodic; euphoric; aphrodisiac; warming; tonic
Physical Applications: PMS; menstrual cramps; digestive cramps; colic; strengthens kidneys and stomach; bronchial asthma; migraine; muscle cramps; dandruff; greasy hair
Subtle Applications: Uplifting; enhances female qualities; deep relaxant; dream work; mood swings; postnatal depression; tension and stress

Precautions: Use sparingly, and never with alcohol — the combination of the two can cause bad dreams and a nasty hangover. Avoid using during the first trimester of pregnancy.

Cinnamon: *Cinnamomum zeylanicum*
Ceylon, India, China

Properties: Antiseptic; antispasmodic; parasiticide; stimulant

Physical Applications: Stimulates cardiovascular system; flu (preventive); impotence; childbirth; lice; scabies

Subtle Applications: Aphrodisiac

Precautions: Do not us undiluted on the skin. High doses can cause skin irritation and convulsions. Avoid during pregnancy. Can be used during labor to stimulate uterine contractions.

Cypress: *Cupressus sempervirens*
France, Spain, Morocco

Properties: Astringent; drainer; antispasmodic

Physical Applications: Water retention; stagnated lymph system; cellulite; edema; bronchial asthma; sore throat; whooping cough; excess perspiration; painful and/or heavy menstrual flow; oily skin; hemorrhoids; bleeding gums; varicose veins; menopause.

Subtle Applications: Longevity; strength; eases irritability; restorative to nervous system

Eucalyptus: *Eucalyptus globulus*
Australia, Spain

Properties: Expectorant; antiseptic; deodorant; decongestant; antibacterial; antiviral; diuretic

Physical Applications: Respiratory problems; draining; throat problems (*australiana*); insect repellent (lice and mosquitoes); fever; flu; bronchitis; cough; sinusitis; urinary tract infections; burns; wounds; cold sores and shingles; rheumatism; muscle aches; intestinal parasites; migraine

Subtle Applications: Invigorating; balancing; purifying; enhances vitality

Fennel: *Foeniculum vulgare*
Spain, North Africa, India

Properties: Diuretic; cleansing; detoxifying

Physical Applications: Nausea; flatulence; sluggish digestion; colic; hiccoughs; painful, scanty periods; menstrual cycle regulation; PMS; water retention; cellulitis; retention of urine; urinary tract infection; menopause; increases milk flow in nursing mothers; relieves congestion of breasts; bruises, tumors; gum infections (gargle, mouthwash)

Precautions: Do not use with children under age six. One of its chemical constituents, Melanthine, can be toxic to small children, though harmless to older children and adults. Should not be used by epileptics.

Frankincense: *Boswellia carteri*
North Africa

Properties: Slows and deepens breath; pulmonary antiseptic

Physical Applications: Coughs; chronic bronchitis; asthma; older skin; wrinkles; urino-genital infections; uterine tonic; heavy periods

Subtle Applications: Meditation; calming; anxiety; breaking links with the past
Can be used during pregnancy.

Geranium: *Pelargonium roseum*
Reunion, France, China

Properties: Cytophylactic; cellular stimulant; antidiabetic; astringent; hemostatic; anti-depressant; antiseptic; diuretic

Physical Applications: Stimulates adrenal cortex; stimulates cell regeneration; regulates hormones; PMS; menopause; fluid retention; cellulitis; stimulates lymphatic and capillary circulation; throat problems; sluggish, oily, or congested skin; contact dermatitis; herpes; sores; burns; congestion of breasts; sore throat; tonsilitis; lice; dry eczema; lumbar pains

Subtle Applications: Invigorating; balancing; rejuvenating; harmonizing; uplifting; anxiety; nervous tension; depression; stress; debility

Grapefruit: *Citrus paradisi*
United States
Properties: Antiseptic; antiviral; antidepressant
Physical Applications: Cellulite; PMS; nervous depression
Subtle Applications: Confidence; positive outlook; "lightening up"
Precautions: Like other citruses, grapefruit should not be used on the skin before going out into the sun, as it may increase photosensitivity.

Helichrysum: *Helichrysum angustifolium, H. italicum*
France, Corsica
Properties: Anti-inflammatory; antispasmodic; antihematoma; mucolytic
Physical Applications: Contusions; sprains; swelling; skin disorders; couperose skin; rhinitis; cough; bronchitis; asthma; allergies; arthritis
Precautions: Use sparingly due to high ketone content.

Jasmine: *Jasminum officinale, J. grandiflorum* (absolute)
India, Egypt, Morocco
Properties: Uterine tonic; aphrodisiac
Physical Applications: PMS; menstrual cramps; frigidity; childbirth; coughs; chest infections; loss of voice; dry or sensitive skin
Subtle Applications: Uplifting; promotes optimism; antidepressant; relaxant; warming; boosts confidence

Juniper berry: *Juniperus communis*

Italy

Properties: Antiseptic; diuretic; tonic; purifying; stimulant; parasiticide

Physical Applications: Slow digestion; flatulence; urinogenital tract infections; cystitis; pyelitis; urinary stones; urine retention (prostate enlargement); leucorrhea; scanty or missed periods; painful or difficult periods; acne; rheumatism; arthritis (related to poor elimination); weeping eczema; psoriasis; dermatitis; canine care: canker, mange, fleas and ticks

Subtle Applications: General debility; psychic purification

Precautions: Do not use if pregnant, or if there is a history of kidney problems.

Lavender: *Lavandula officinalis, L. angustifolia, L. vera*

France, Tasmania

(For a full profile of this most versatile and useful of all essential oils, see Chapter Two.)

Properties: Balancing; antiseptic; cytophilactic; rejuvenating; antispasmodic; sedative; antifungal

Physical Applications: Burns; wounds; cell regeneration; skin conditions; promotes healing, prevents scarring; acne/oily skin; sensitive/inflamed skin; eczema; insect bites; insect repellent; respiratory conditions; sinusitis; sharp pains; muscle aches; rheumatism; sciatica; arthritis; painful or scanty periods; leucorrhea; childbirth; colic; childhood infections, fretfulness; heart palpitations; high blood pressure; athlete's foot; ringworm

Subtle Applications: Calming; soothing; regulates sleep patterns; balancing; nervous exhaustion; hysteria; manic depression; mood swings

Lemon: *Citrus limonum*

United States

Properties: Stimulant; tonic; stomachic; stimulates production of white corpuscles; hemostatic; bactericide; counteracts acidity in body; astringent

Physical Applications: Oily skin; wrinkles; controls secretions; blood fluidifier; bronchitis; head colds; flu; fever; gastric conditions; vomiting; bleeding gums; nosebleeds; broken capillaries; varicose veins; high blood pressure; corns, warts, verrucas; insect repellent (clothes moths, ants)

Subtle Applications: Refreshing; optimistic; promotes fearlessness; strengthening; anti-aging

Precautions: Like most citrus oils, lemon can cause skin irritation and increase photosensitivity. Use concentrations of less than 1%. In a bath, no more than two to three drops.

Lemongrass: *Cymbopogon citratu*
India, Madagascar, Guatemala
Properties: Antiseptic; bactericide; parasiticide; tonic; stimulant; detoxifying
Physical Applications: Colds; fever; digestion; headache; PMS; cramps; dizziness; deodorant; sweaty feet; oily skin; insect repellent; lice
Subtle Applications: Stress; balancing
Precautions: Use sparingly, in dilution only — potential skin irritant.

Mandarin: *Citrus nobilis, C. madurensis, C. reticulata var. mandarin*
Italy
Properties: Sedative; antispasmodic; light hypnotic
Physical Applications: Digestive problems; children's and elderly complaints, such as stomach upsets, burps, hiccoughs and insomnia; stretch marks (preventive)
Subtle Applications: Overexcitement; anguish; relaxation; good dreams

Marjoram: *Origanum majorana*
France, Germany
Properties: Analgesic, antispasmodic; sedative; anaphrodisiac
Physical Applications: Bronchitis; asthma; colds; tickly throat and chest; insomnia;

dilates arteries (reducing strain on heart); muscle pain/exhaustion; rheumatism; arthritis; colic; intestinal cramps

Subtle Applications: Grief; loneliness; mental instabililty

Precautions: Overuse of marjoram can be somewhat addictive and have a dulling effect on the emotions.

Myrrh: *Commiphora molmol*
Somalia

Properties: Anti-inflammative; antiseptic; antifungal; astringent; expectorant; tonic

Physical Applications: Bronchitis; coughs; colds; infected wounds; cold sores; acne; dermatitis; athlete's foot; gum problems; diarrhea; sore throat

Subtle Applications: Meditation; opening of psychic centers

Precautions: Do not use during pregnancy.

Neroli: *Citrus aurantium, C. vulgaris*
Morocco, France

Properties: Antiseptic; antispasmodic; antidepressant; sedative; rejuvenating; aphrodisiac

Physical Applications: Dry/sensitive/inflamed skin; aging skin; diarrhea (from nervous tension)

Subtle Applications: Anxiety; shock; hysteria; nervous tension; insomnia

Precautions: Don't use this oil for relaxation if any degree of alertness will be required of you, such as while driving or at work.

Niaouli: *Melaleuca viridiflora, M. quinquenervia viridiflora*
Madagascar, New Caledonia

Properties: Antiseptic; stimulant; aids in tissue growth; analgesic; vermifuge

Physical Applications: Oily skin; bronchitis; flu; whooping cough; runny nose; sinusitis; earache; cystitis; urethritis; rheumatism; intestinal parasites; burns; laryngitis

Orange: *Citrus aurantium, var. amara; C. vulgaris; C. bigardia* (all bitter orange) *Citrus aurantium var. dulcis; C. sinensis* (sweet orange)
United States, Israel
Properties: Antidepressant; antispasmodic; stomachic; sedative (mild)
Physical Applications: Sluggish lymph system; digestive problems; constipation; chronic diarrhea
Subtle Applications: Calming; cheerful; uplifting
Precautions: *Use sparingly. Like other citruses, more than a few drops can cause skin irritation.*

Palmarosa: *Cymbopogon martini*
Guatemala
Properties: Antiseptic; cellular stimulant; hydrating
Physical Applications: Wrinkles; skin imbalance; acne (balances sebum production)
Subtle Applications: Calming; refreshing; uplifting

Peppermint: *Mentha piperita*
United States, England
Properties: Antiseptic; digestive; tonic; stimulant; antispasmodic; analgesic; cephalic; parasiticide
Physical Applications: Digestive upset; headache; fever; fainting; colic; diarrhea; vomiting; colds; flu; nausea; gas; bloating; heartburn; seasickness; scabies; asthma; pest repellent (mosquitoes, gnats, vermin)
Subtle Applications: Clarity; shock (emergency treatment); mental fatigue
Precautions: *Use sparingly, can cause intense cold or tingling sensations on the skin. Do not use with homeopathics or store near homeopathic remedies, as peppermint is said to neutralize their effects. Avoid using at bedtime, or over extended periods, as heavy use of peppermint can be over-stimulating and disrupt sleep patterns.*

Pine: *Pinus maritimus, P. sylvestris*
Russia, Finland

Properties: Pulmonary and urinary antiseptic; expectorant; rubefacient; hepatic

Physical Applications: Colds; catarrh; sore throat; sinus problems; flu; circulation; rheumatic pain; muscular pain; kidney problems; deodorant; sweaty feet; scabies; lice

Subtle Applications: Warming; comforting; stress release

Precautions: *Dwarf pine,* Pinus pumilio, *is a hazardous oil and should not be used for purposes of aromatherapy. Use pine essential oil sparingly, and always in dilution, as too much can cause skin irritation.*

Ravensara: *Ravensara aromatica*
Madagascar

Properties: Antiseptic; antiviral; expectorant; neurotonic

Physical Applications: Flu; grippe; zona (shingles); mononucleosis

Subtle Applications: Insomnia

Rose: *Rosa centifolia, R. damascena, R. gallica*
France, Morocco, Bulgaria, Turkey

Properties: General tonic; cleansing; purifying; regulating; cell regenerator; moisturizer

Physical Applications: Uterus and female reproductive system; uterine prolapse; tendency to miscarriage; eczema, wrinkles, dryness, puffiness, pore congestion, aging/ sensitive skin

Subtle Applications: Gentle but potent antidepressant; emotional imbalances manifesting in reproductive or sexual disturbances; postnatal depression; emotional shock; grief; tension; sadness; low self-esteem; revitalizing; opening the heart

Rosemary: *Rosmarinus officinalis*
Tunisia, Spain

Properties: General stimulant; cephalic; cardiotonic; rubefacient; antiseptic; aphrodisiac; parasiticide

Physical Applications: Central nervous system disorders; lowering cholesterol levels in blood; respiratory problems; muscle pains; weakness in children; rheumatism; arthritis; wounds, sores, burns; muscle pain; scalp conditions; dandruff; hair loss; dry skin; acne; rinse for dark hair

Subtle Applications: Fatigue; mental strain; memory aid; anemia; general recuperation

Precaution: Use sparingly. High concentrations of rosemary can bring on epileptic fits.

Rosewood: *Aniba roseaodora*
Brazil

Properties: Cellular stimulant; emollient; antibacterial; deodorant; tonic; analgesic

Physical Applications: Dry, sensitive skin; pimples; acne; wrinkles; scars

Subtle Applications: Soothing; euphoric; calming; steadying; uplifting

Sandalwood: *Santalum album*
India (Mysore)

Properties: Urinary tract disinfectant; pulmonary disinfectant; sedative; antiseptic; aphrodisiac

Physical Applications: Genitourinary infections; dry, dehydrated skin; sensitive/inflamed skin; eczema; acne; oily skin (antiseptic); wrinkles; dry, persistent coughs; chronic bronchitis; shaving rash; impotence

Subtle Applications: Aphrodisiac; relaxant; psychospiritual stimulation; meditation; antidepressant; awakens kundalini; centering (apply a drop to the third eye); confusion; fear; stress

Tangerine: *Citrus reticulata*
United States

Properties: Antiseptic; antispasmodic

Physical Applications: Digestive problems; children's and elderly complaints, such as stomach upsets, burps, hiccups

Subtle Applications: Cheerful; uplifting

Precautions: Like all citrus oils, it should not be used before going out in the sun, as it may cause increased photosensitivity. High concentrations may also cause irritation to sensitive skin, so use it sparingly. Safe to use during pregnancy.

Tea Tree: *Melaleuca alternifolia*
Australia

Properties: Antiviral; antifungal; anti-infectious; antibacterial; immunostimulant

Physical Applications: Candida/yeast; herpes; mouth and gum irritations; athlete's foot; fungal infections; wound-healing; dandruff; sinus congestion; colds, flu; infectious childhood diseases; cold sores; shingles; chicken pox; warts; verrucas; pimples; acne; preoperative; insect repellent

Precautions: Use sparingly, and in dilution— can cause irritation on sensitive skin.

Thyme: *Thymus vulgaris*
Spain

Properties: Antiseptic; mucolytic; cytophilactic; vermifuge; antibacterial; diuretic

Physical Applications: Strengthening immune system; bedwetting (thyme tea); cellulitis; circulation; digestive stimulant; intestinal worms (roundworm, threadworm, tapeworm); colds, coughs; sore throats; bronchitis; flu; hair loss; mouth and gum infections; urinary tract and bladder infections; low blood pressure; rheumatism; insect bites; lice, scabies

Subtle Applications: Fatigue; depression; insomnia; convalescence

Precautions: Thymus vulgaris *must be used sparingly, since it can cause skin irritation. Better to use it in inhalations and room sprays. Try thyme linalol for anything coming into contact with the skin.*

Ylang-Ylang: *Cananga odorata*

Comoro Islands

Properties: Relaxant; euphoric; vasodilator; antidepressant; sedative; aphrodisiac

Physical Applications: Oily skin; dry skin; hair growth; impotence; frigidity; high blood pressure; tachycardia; high blood pressure; balances production of sebum

Subtle Applications: Sexual response; anger; frustration; fright; insomnia

Precautions: *Overuse can cause headaches and nausea.*

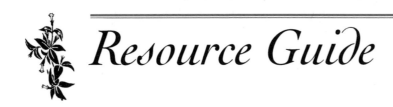

Resource Guide

Essential Oils

The following are reputable suppliers of essential oils. Call for catalogs and ordering information, or for a store location near you.

Aroma Vera 1-800-669-9514
Oshadi 1-800-933-1008
Time Laboratories 1-208-232-5250

Carrier Oils

An excellent source for high-quality carrier and specialty oils, including jojoba and *Rosa rubignosa*.

Janca Naturals 1-602-833-4940

Essential Oil Products

Just because it says "aromatherapy" on the label is no guarantee that you're getting a product made with authentic essential oils. The following companies can be relied upon to supply quality products using pure essential oils. Look for them in your local health food store or bath and body boutique, or call the company to find a retail location near you.

Aromaland 1-800-933-5267
Essential oil blends and diffusors

Aroma Vera 1-800-669-9514
Essential oils, aromatherapy bath and beauty products

Aroma West 1-310-391-0787
Essential oil blends, bath oils and sprays

Carol Corio Quality of Life Associates 1-800-688-8343
Aromatherapy diffusors and products

Crystalessence Aromatherapy 1-800-688-8343
Aromatherapy candles and body care products

Essential Aromatics 1-805-640-1300
Aromatherapy candles, bath salts, massage oils, handcrafted in Ojai, California

Essential Elements 1-415-621-9881
Aromatherapy bath salts, shower gels, shampoos, sprays

Mon Jardinet 1-212-877-3044
Aromatherapy bath and body care products

Neal's Yard 1-415-621-1075
Essential oils and aromatherapy products

Original Swiss Aromatics 1-415-479-9121
Essential oils, aromatherapy bath, beauty and massage products

Oshadi 1-800-933-1008
Complete line of essential oils and aromatherapy products

Quan Yin Essentials 1-707-431-0529
Aromatherapy bath salts, massage oils, and pillow sprays

Time Laboratories 1-208-232-5250
Essential oils and aromatherapy products

Tisserand Aromatherapy 1-707-769-5120
Essential oils and aromatherapy products

wives tales-1-800-955-8253
Aromatherapy for kids, aromatherapy for women, bath and body products

Further Education
Aromatherapy Seminars 1-800-677-2368
Michael Scholes, Introductory Through Certification-Level Courses

Pacific Institute of Aromatherapy 1-415-479-9121
Dr. Kurt Schnaubelt, Certification and Correspondence Course

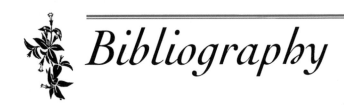

Bibliography

Ackerman, Diane. *A Natural History of the Senses*
New York, Random House, 1990

Bremness, Lesley. *The Complete Book of Herbs*
New York, Viking Studio Books, 1988

Calder, Nigel. *Timescale*
New York, Viking Press, 1983

Campbell, H. J. *The Pleasure Areas: A New Theory of Behavior*
London, Eyre Methuen Ltd., 1973

Dadd, Debra Lynn. *Nontoxic, Natural and Earthwise*
Los Angeles, Jeremy P. Tarcher, Inc., 1990

Curtis, Susan and Fraser, Romy. *Natural Healing for Women*
London, Pandora, 1991

Davis, Patricia. *Aromatherapy: An A-Z*
England, C. W. Daniel, 1988

Dethlefsen, Thorwald. *The Healing Power of Illness*
Great Britain, Element Books, 1990

Fox, Helen Morgenthau. *Gardening with Herbs for Flavor and Fragrance*
New York, Dover, 1933/1970

Frawley, David and Lad, Vasant. *The Yoga of Herbs*
Santa Fe, New Mexico, Lotus Press, 1986

Hutchens, Alma R. *Indian Herbalogy of North America*
Ontario, Canada, Merco, 1969/1986

Jackson, Judith. *Scentual Touch: A Personal Guide to Aromatherapy*
New York, Henry Holt & Co., 1986

Marian, Alda and Jangl, James Francis. *Ancient Legends of Healing Herbs*
Prisma Press, 1987

Jones, Julia and Deer, Barbara. *The Country Diary of Garden Lore*
New York, Summit Books, 1989

Lavabre, Marcel. *Aromatherapy Workbook*
Rochester, Vermont, Healing Arts Press, 1990

Lima, Patrick. *The Harrowsmith Illustrated Book of Herbs*
Ontario, Canada, Camden House, 1986

Maury, Marguerite. *Marguerite Maury's Guide to Aromatherapy*
England, C. W. Daniel, 1989

Messegue, Maurice. *Of People and Plants*
Rochester, Vermont, Healing Arts Press, 1973

Metcalfe, Johanna. *Herbs and Aromatherapy*
London, Webb and Bower, 1989

Montagu, Ashley. *Touching: The Human Significance of the Skin*
New York, Harper & Row, 1986

Ramsey, Teresa. *Baby's First Massage*

Rohde, Eleanour Sinclair. *The Old English Herbals*
New York, Dover, 1922/1971

Rose, Jeanne. *Jeanne Rose's Kitchen Cosmetics*
Berkeley, California, North Atlantic Books, 1990

Rudolfsky, Bernard. *Now I Lay Me Down to Eat*
New York, Anchor Books, 1980

Ryman, Daniele. *The Aromatherapy Handbook*
Woodstock, New York, Beekman Publishers, 1990

Schnaubelt, Kurt. *Aromatherapy Course*
San Rafael, California, Pacific Institute

Scott, Julian. *Natural Medicine for Children*
New York, Avon Books, 1990

Sinclair, Marybetts. *Massage for Healthier Children*
Oakland, California, Wingbow Press, 1992

Stockwell, Christine. *Nature's Pharmacy*
London, Century, 1988

Stoddart, D. Michael. *The Scented Ape: The Biology and Culture of Human Odor*
Cambridge, England, Cambridge University Press, 1990

Tenney, Louise. *Today's Herbal Health*
Provo, Utah, Woodland Books, 1983

Tierra, Michael. *The Way of Herbs*
New York, Pocket Books, 1983

Tisserand, Maggie. *Aromatherapy for Women*
Rochester, Vermont, Healing Arts Press, 1985

Tisserand, Robert. *Aromatherapy: To Heal and Tend the Body*
Santa Fe, New Mexico, Lotus Press, 1988

Tisserand, Robert. *The Essential Oil Safety Data Manual*
England, Tisserand Aromatherapy Institute, 1990

Tobe, John H. *Proven Herbal Remedies*
Canada, Provoker Press, 1969

Valnet, Jean, M.D. *The Practice of Aromatherapy*
New York, Destiny Books, 1982

Vigarello, Georges. *Concepts of Cleanliness*
Cambridge, England, Cambridge University Press, 1988

Walker, Barbara G. *The Woman's Encyclopedia of Myths and Secrets*
San Francisco, Harper San Francisco, 1983

Worwood, Valerie. *The Fragrant Pharmacy*
  London, Macmillan, 1990

Editors of Sunset Books and Magazine, *Sunset Western Garden Book*
  Menlo Park, California, Sunset Publishing, 1991